DR. A

the ***end*** *of*
DIABETES
MELLITUS

Discover how to ***be free*** from symptoms,
medications, and complications
in ***less than 21 days***

WITHOUT MEDICATIONS

100% EFFECTIVE AND NATURAL

AQS
ACADEMY

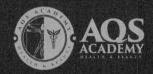

The End of Diabetes Mellitus
2024, Alden J. Quesada, MD
ISBN: 979-88-84-68475-1
Library of Congress Control Number (LCCN):
20229007278

■

■

COVER AND LAYOUT
Jonatas Ilustre

■

1st Edition: March 2024

International Cataloging-in-Publication Data
(Câmara Brasileira do Livro, SP, Brazil)

Quesada, Alden J.
    The End of Diabetes Mellitus: discover how to be free from symptoms, medications,
and complications in less than 21 days with the only 100% natural method: no need
for medications, without leaving your home, quickly and safely / Alden J. Quesada.
- Presidente Venceslau, SP: Self-Published, 2023.

    Bibliography.
    ISBN 979-88-84-68475-1

    1. Diabetes mellitus. 2. Diabetes - Care and treatment. 3. Diabetes -
Daygnosis 4. Diabetes - Diet therapy 5. Diabetes - Prevention I. Title.

	CDD-616.462
23-177698	NLM-WK-810

Indices for systematic catalog:
Diabetes Mellitus: Medicine 616.462
Aline Grazielle Benitez - Librarian - CRB-1/3129

the *end* of
DIABETES
MELLITUS

DEDICATION

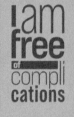

the *end* of
**DIABETES
MELLITUS**

DEDICATION

To our Creator, for the blessing of knowledge and the calling to help others.

To Rafael A. Milanés Santana. His boundless passion for true medicine, the kind that heals, and his close friendship with my father, were the source of inspiration for me to become a naturopathic doctor and today have the opportunity to help thousands of people.

A tight hug wherever you may be.

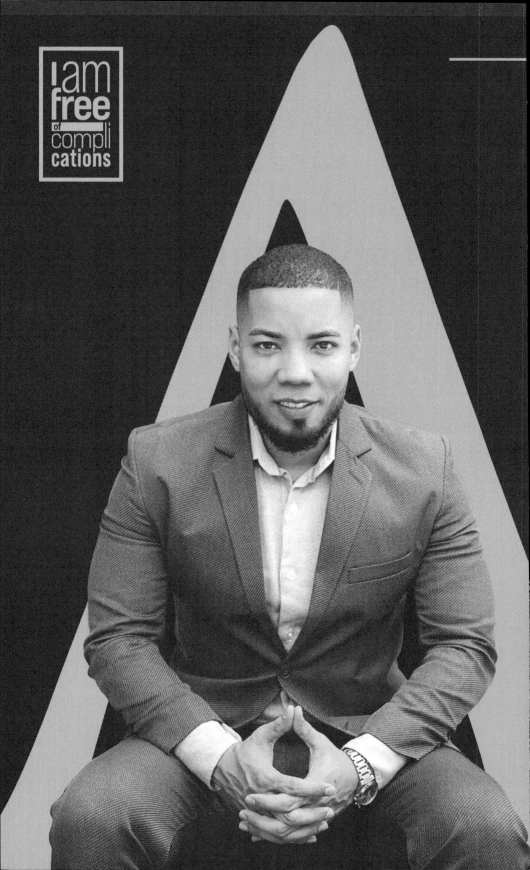

ACKNOW LEDGMENTS

In this book, whose content has already saved thousands of lives across four continents, I first want to thank you, who seek every day the true solution for your health problems, who do not accept watching your symptoms worsen with each passing day and feel the need to take more medications because someone told you it was the only thing you could do.

I am eternally grateful to you, who are nonconformist and wish to be free of symptoms, medications, risks, and complications. You are my greatest inspiration.

I also dedicate words of gratitude to my family, who has to "endure" my absences so that I can study, structure, write, and validate my treatments in practice.

Without a doubt, it is a challenge for them, and for me...

Lastly, I thank all my patients, especially those who have shared their testimonials with me. You cannot imagine the joy it brings me whenever I receive a message, a photo, or a video, where you share your progress and how you were freed from diabetes mellitus.

To all, a tight hug.

#iamfreeofcomplications

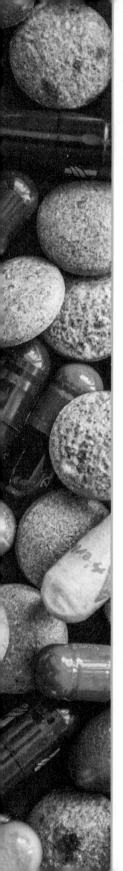

Why you should read this

BOOK

Have you ever asked yourself why you're experiencing more and more symptoms and need to take an increasing amount of medications?

Unfortunately, Diabetes Mellitus (DM) is a threat that you simply cannot afford to ignore.

This silent disease affects and limits the lives of people of all ages and origins, indiscriminately.

Right now, as you read these words, dozens of stealthy symptoms, devastating limitations, and both acute and chronic complications are lurking in the shadows, ready to burst into your life.

SHOCKING FACTS

According to the World Health Organization (WHO), DM ranks among the top causes of death worldwide.

Sadly, each year, millions of people globally fall victim to this disease.

The statistics are disturbing, not to say disheartening, and the reality is deeply concerning.

Worldwide figures provided by the World Diabetes Foundation indicate that:

- Every 7 seconds, a person dies from DM complications.

- As reported by the International Diabetes Federation Atlas, in 2021, 6.7 million people worldwide died due to this disease.

- The risk of individuals with DM developing a foot ulcer is 34%.

- Every 20 seconds, a limb is amputated on a person with DM.

- It is the leading cause of blindness in individuals aged 40 to 74, lower limb amputations, and chronic kidney disease.

- It is the second leading cause of disability in the region, only preceded by ischemic heart disease.

- DM triples the risk of death from cardiovascular diseases, kidney disease, or cancer.

These figures aren't mere numbers; they represent shattered lives and crushed dreams, and there's a significant chance that if you don't take the correct steps, you may someday become part of these grim statistics.

Until today, you've done everything "right":

You took the medications you were told to, attended countless doctor's appointments—where often you weren't truly heard and were mistreated—underwent numerous tests, and never saw any improvement. On the contrary, you've only seen your condition worsen day by day, as you spend your money on medications, doctors, etc., while your health and vitality continue to wane.

BUT HERE'S THE GOOD NEWS:

You still have the opportunity to conquer this disease!

In the pages of this book, you will discover a powerful, 100% effective method that—if applied with discipline and persistence—will definitively reverse the damage caused by diabetes mellitus.

In the upcoming chapters, the path towards health, vitality, and the freedom that you've undoubtedly been searching for tirelessly will be unveiled.

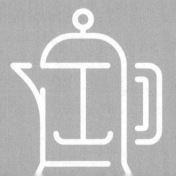

With each passing day that the damage caused by this disease isn't reversed, the risk of acute and chronic complications increases. You can't afford to wait any longer!

Don't risk becoming another statistic. It's time to retake control of your destiny and change the course of your life before it's too late.

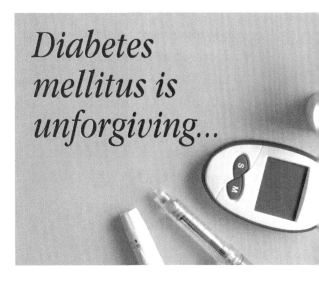

Diabetes mellitus is unforgiving...

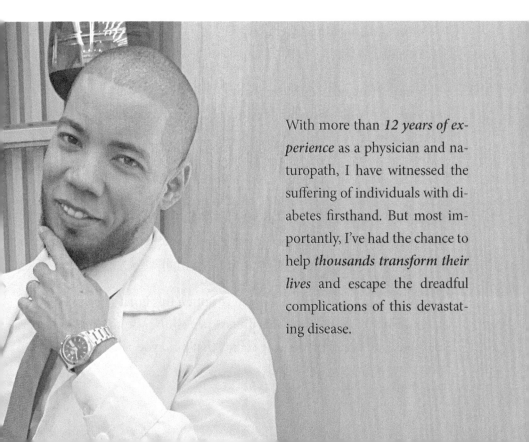

With more than *12 years of experience* as a physician and naturopath, I have witnessed the suffering of individuals with diabetes firsthand. But most importantly, I've had the chance to help *thousands transform their lives* and escape the dreadful complications of this devastating disease.

Now, I want you to close your eyes and imagine you're ten years older, and your health situation has continued to deteriorate just as it has until now.

What would you tell yourself?

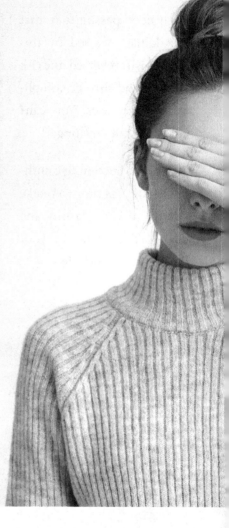

How would you feel if, looking back on your life, you had to regret not having decided to read this book and apply the simple yet powerful recommendations I'm sharing with you here?

The opportunity is right in front of you, but only you can decide whether to seize it or let it pass by.

Diabetes mellitus doesn't forgive inaction, especially not the thought that *"it won't happen to me"*; the consequences of failing to take control of your health can be catastrophic.

However, I am confident that if you've gotten this far, it's because your desire to be free from this disease is pushing you to explore new paths to break the terrible chains that bind you and prevent you from living life to the fullest.

This book—or rather, the content I share within it—has the power to dramatically change your destiny, just as it has already helped thousands. It's simply a matter of making the right choice.

You don't have to suffer endlessly with this disease. I invite you to accept my help and *live the full life you deserve.*

By following the recommendations in this book, you'll discover how simple it is to take back control of your health and live the life you're entitled to— we have no time to lose...

Turn the page, again and again, as the most closely guarded secrets to liberating yourself from the shadow of diabetes are revealed.

Your life is at stake, and I know you will make the right choice.

*the **end** of*
**DIABETES
MELLITUS**

ADVICE

from Dr. Quesada

1. Read the entire book, take notes on your questions, and consult anything you find difficult to understand on the Internet, with your family, or preferably with your doctor.

2. Commit to yourself, and to your family, to follow the instructions in this book for at least 30 days without making excuses.

3. If you do not have one, purchase a Glucometer and test strips to monitor your blood sugar levels.

4. Buy the foods needed to prepare the recipes indicated for specific times of the day.

5. Start carrying out the Daily Recommendations, no matter if you don't have all the products, begin with the Normoglycemic Tea and the Cucumber Juice, then gradually incorporate the rest of the recommendations.

6. Avoid eating foods that are classified as prohibited.

7. Perform the three recommended daily checks to be aware of your progress:

   - Blood Sugar Control.
   - Daily Recommendations Control.
   - Symptom Evolution Control.

Lastly, always keep this book close to you as if it were your second Bible because by mastering, and putting into practice, the recommendations I propose, I am confident that you will be free of symptoms, medications, risks, and complications, ensuring the life you deserve and that your family deserves.

A Big Hug,
Dr. Alden J. Quesada

The Quarrel That
CHANGED HISTORY

THE BACTERIA [VS] THE "TERRAIN"
LOUIS PASTEUR [VS] CLAUDE BERNARD

In the 19th century, a momentous scientific debate took place in the field of medicine.

On one side, Louis Pasteur, the renowned French scientist, argued that *"disease was due to the entry of microorganisms (viruses and bacteria) into the body, which altered the function of organs and tissues."*

On the other side, Claude Bernard, also a French scientist but less famous than Pasteur, maintained that *"disease was produced by a defective or weak state of the terrain—our body."*

The majority of scientific currents supported Pasteur's thesis that the microorganism was more important than *"the terrain—the state of the body."*

However, to everyone's surprise, shortly before dying, Pasteur acknowledged with his now-famous phrase that Claude Bernard was right: *"The agent is nothing. The terrain is everything."*

AUTHOR'S NOTE:

I read this article for the first time when I was 17 years old at Professor Rafael Milanés Santana's house, and he had titled it somewhat like this: "The quarrel that changed history."

At that time, I knew absolutely nothing about medicine, but my admiration for him, who worked together with my father, grew enormously to the point that it became a powerful incentive for me to delve into the wonderful world of medicine and natural therapies.

Today it is proven that the most important thing is the state of the body, homeostasis, balance, functioning, and that is why, when we stimulate the body's detoxification process in the right way, we can reverse symptoms, decrease medication doses, and avoid complications from most diseases.

Thank you, Milanés, for the wealth of knowledge you shared with me, a tight hug...

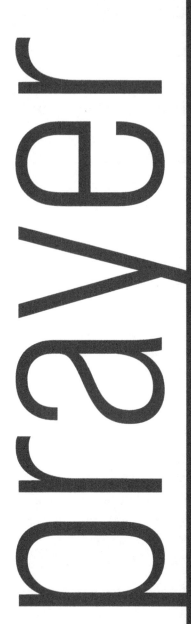

prayer

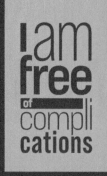

I am free of compli cations

Special Request

Now, I ask you to pay close attention, because I am going to make a special request.

Something I want to become part of your life and that you are absolutely sure will bring you a change and a freedom you never imagined.

Every day, upon waking and before going to sleep, say the *"I Am Free of Complications"* Prayer. It is very powerful and will generate a state of well-being and transformative confidence.

This prayer serves as a reminder of your commitment to your health and your will to live many years, free of symptoms, risks, and complications.

How to do it?

Each morning, before getting out of bed, and before closing your eyes to sleep, repeat the *Prayer.*

I recommend that you set a reminder on your phone so as not to forget to do the Prayer.

My Prayer

I [name], declare, with all the strength of my heart and supported by my desire to live free of symptoms, medications, risks, and complications, that I will apply the method "The End of Diabetes Mellitus."

The Method will accompany me throughout my life and will provide me with the tranquility and security that I deserve and that my family deserves.

I declare that I Am Free of Complications
I Can. I deserve it. I achieve it.

#iamfreeofcomplications

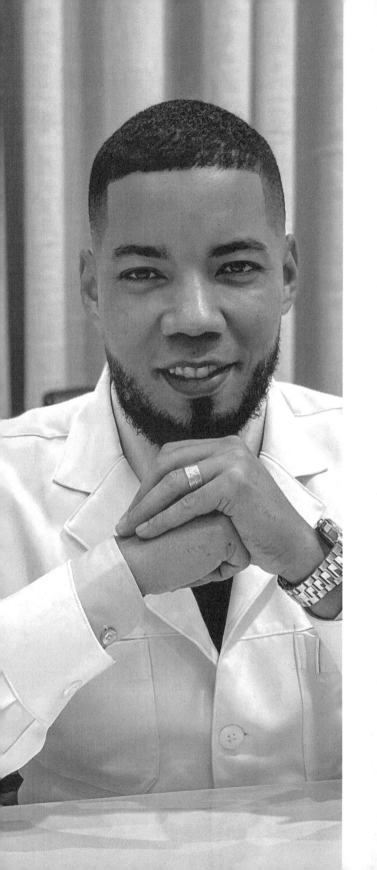

Alden J. Quesada

After losing several of his most beloved relatives to complications from diabetes mellitus, Dr. Alden J. Quesada has dedicated the last 12 years of his professional life to helping people with this disease.

Dr. Quesada, as he is known to his students and patients, is the creator of methods such as *"The End of Diabetes Mellitus," "Diabetes Mellitus: The End of Complications,"* and *"Overcoming Diabetes Mellitus in the Family."*

He has transformed and saved the lives of thousands of daybetic individuals in over 71 countries (including Brazil, the United States, Spain, Mexico, Colombia, and Chile), helping them to be free from symptoms, medications, risks, and complications through the application of his natural treatment protocols.

A professor, scientific researcher, writer, and lover of good music and puppies, especially the Golden Retriever breed, he initially studied Universal History.

Interestingly, he began delving into the world of natural therapies in his adolescence, influenced by his father, who was a renowned naturopathic physician.

Following the death of his father, he decided to restart his studies in Medicine, following in the footsteps and honoring the legacy of his progenitor, graduating in Medicine in 2011 and specializing in Cardiology in 2016 (Cuba).

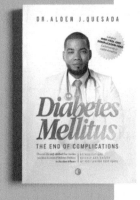

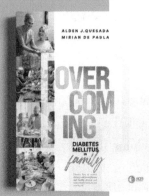

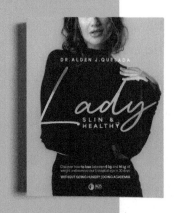

With work experience in four Latin American countries, including the Venezuelan Amazon and Cusco (Peru), he has witnessed and lived with the poverty and lack of health resources for the majority of the sick, experiencing the pain and suffering of daybetic individuals daily.

His research on obesity, diabetes mellitus, and associated diseases has been published in various congresses and scientific journals.

In Dr. Quesada's training as a cardiologist and naturopath, several prestigious figures have participated, such as his father, Dr. Eulogio Quesada, Dr. Delfín Rodríguez Leyva, a world leader in the research of nutraceuticals, and professor Rafael Milanés Santana, a reference authority on the medicinal use of plants and macrobiotics.

He has also received national and international awards for his contribution to the study and control of chronic diseases with 100% effective methods, free of risks and side effects.

Professor Quesada's mission is to reduce mortality related to complications from diabetes mellitus and cardiovascular diseases.

To achieve this goal, he founded the AQS Institute of Natural Therapies and the largest and only community of daybetic individuals in Latin America who are free from symptoms, risks, and complications.

My mission is that no more lives are lost due to complications from this disease, and that is why I idealized, created, and care with all my energy for the movement:

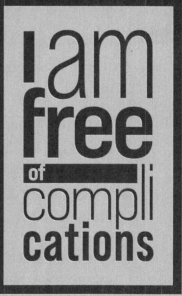

I am free of compli cations

PRO LO GUE

Are natural therapies the vehicle to treat diabetes mellitus?

In the book *"The End of Diabetes mellitus,"* Dr. Alden J. Quesada introduces a novel method that opens new ways to treat a complex medical condition considered a major cause of heart attacks, strokes, renal failure, lower limb amputations, and blindness.

Dr. Quesada is a renowned cardiologist trained in treating cardayc and metabolic diseases.

He transforms his experience as a brilliant cardiologist into a new dimension of patient management that avoids the use of Western medicine to treat diabetes mellitus successfully.

Modern treatments for diabetes mellitus are expensive and carry significant side effects.

There is a proven association between diabetes mellitus and heart diseases, and Professor Quesada's experience has allowed the introduction of a new method that focuses on the beneficial effects of natural therapies in treating diabetes, with the potential to positively impact millions of lives worldwide.

Delfín Rodríguez Leyva

MD, Ph.D, FRCPC, FAHA.

*Professor of Cardiology
MHC. Toronto. ON. Canadá*

The proposed method, scientifically verified by Professor Quesada, originates from a deep understanding of the physiology and pathophysiology of this condition and leverages the use of plants, fruits, and natural products to modify the internal signaling of the disease in our body.

The use of such innovative therapy allows treating diabetes in a 100% natural way and aims to control the disease and prevent its complications.

The proposed pathways for carrying out body detoxification are:

1. Provision of the nutrients necessary for proper cellular functioning.

2. Stimulation of the natural mechanisms of elimination of toxic substances from the body, such as free radicals and end products of glycation.

Patients, as well as medical professionals, will find in this book an excellent source of knowledge to control diabetes and prevent its complications.

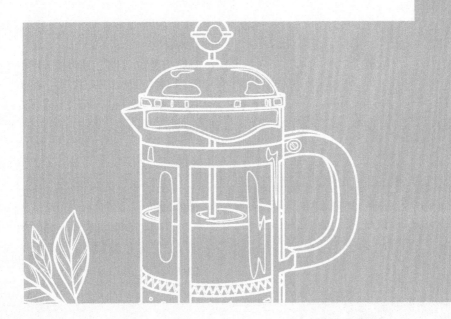

SUMMARY

eu sou
livre
de
compli
cações

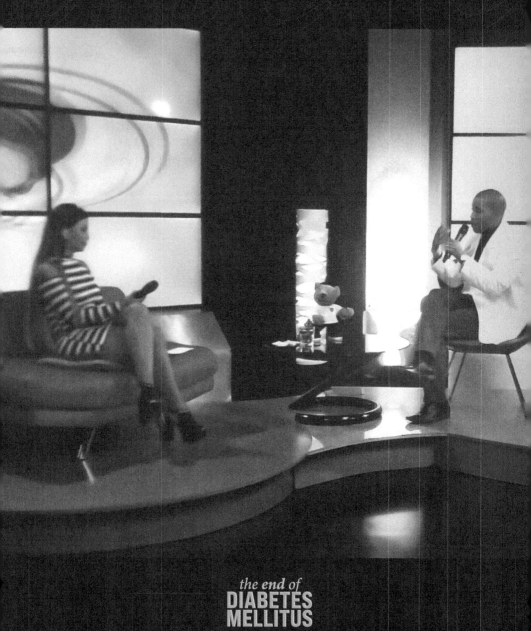

the end of
DIABETES
MELLITUS

INTRO
DUCTION

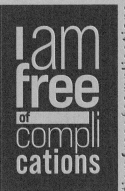

#iamfreeofcomplications

@draldenquesada.es

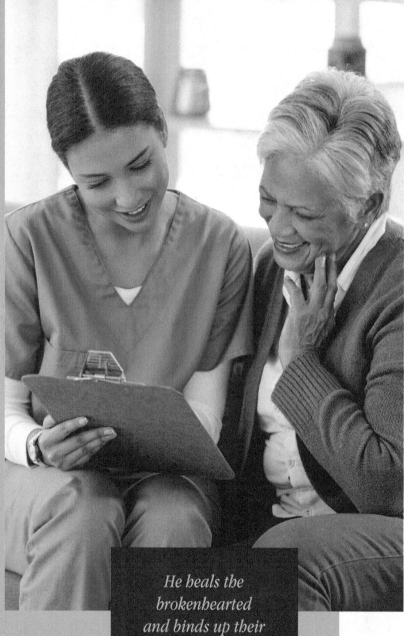

the end of
**DIABETES
MELLITUS**

*He heals the
brokenhearted
and binds up their
wounds.*

PSALM 147:3

Have you ever felt that diabetes affects not just your body but also your soul, distances you from your dreams, and destroys your interpersonal relationships?

The fight against diabetes mellitus has been a challenging and painful battle for millions of people worldwide.

———————

My experience with diabetes mellitus began long before I studied medicine and in the worst way possible - within my family - as two of my cousins, both brothers, had this disease. I do not share their names out of respect for their memory.

The older one, E.Q., gradually lost his vision until he was completely blind, and then the complications came one after another: gangrene of the feet requiring progressive amputation, cardiovascular disorders, etc.

My other cousin, the younger one to whom I was particularly close and admired, was one of the most beloved people in his small town called Minas.

I have many memories of visiting him frequently on weekends. Getting up early to go for cow's milk, straight from the *"udder of the cow,"* which, along with the freshly processed country cheese and freshly baked bread, were part of our morning ritual.

I never knew anyone more family-oriented and endearing than L.Q., but life and the mismanagement of diabetes mellitus would also play a cruel trick on him.

#iamfreeofcomplications

Years later, while I was studying medicine, on a very hot morning as I was entering the hospital where I was to see my patients, by one of those capricious "coincidences" of life, L.Q.'s wife was crying at the entrance of the Medical Emergency Room.

When she saw me coming, she walked towards me and gave me a hug: *"L.Q. died of a heart attack."*

I can still feel the pain I experienced at that moment; someone like him did not deserve to go so soon.

The image of my father, who was also a doctor and, of course, the family doctor, explaining to him how he should take care of his diabetes and how he should take his medications diligently so that what happened to his brother E.Q. did not happen to him, came to my mind.

Today I can say that it was not diabetes mellitus that ended the lives of my two cousins. It was ignorance, with a significant dose of indiscipline known as self-sabotage.

They did not follow the dietary recommendations and were even less aware of the beneficial effects of natural therapies to control and reverse kidney, neurological, and cardiovascular damage.

My family was never the same without the joy of E.Q. and L.Q. I will always be grateful to them because they were extraordinary human beings.

How I wish I had had the experience I have now in treating and reversing the damage of diabetes back then!

The third significant impact related to diabetes mellitus and its unfair way of snatching lives occurred during my stay in the Venezuelan Amazon, in 2010, while on medical duty at the Comprehensive Daygnostic Medical Center in Puerto Ayacucho.

It was already nightfall, and the shift had been quiet until that moment, but we had no idea that everything was about to change in an instant.

Suddenly we noticed that the ambulance was entering the center at high speed, and when the paramedic opened the doors, the first thing he said was: *"this girl is very serious."*

I will never forget those words...

I don't remember the name of the young woman, but her mother told us she was 16 years old and daygnosed with Type 1 Diabetes Mellitus.

She was insulin-dependent, and for 2 days in the place where they lived, a town called Maroa, there was no insulin nor way to get out because the river was swollen, and the boats couldn't reach them.

The presence of an acute complication of diabetes called ketoacidosis was evident.

The story of the lack of insulin, the respiratory pattern, oral breath, and laboratory tests confirmed the daygnosis.

We quickly made the appropriate corrections with agility and an adrenaline rush I don't remember ever having experi-

#iamfreeofcomplications

enced before, and in less than 2 hours, the young woman was out of danger, hydrated, with recovery of consciousness, and normalization of clinical parameters.

She had responded very well to the treatment, and we were happy and confident with her progress. She was alive by a miracle!

Since she was a minor, it was our responsibility, after stabilizing her, to refer her to the only public hospital in the city, José Gregorio, and so we did.

What we didn't imagine was that something terrible would happen in the next few hours, and we never anticipated it...

The next day, during the handover of the shift, we were informed that the young woman had died in the hospital. At that moment, the cause of death for us was obvious: lack of adequate medical attention.

I can't imagine the pain of the young woman's mother at that moment because, when she left our center, she said goodbye to us happily and thanked us for the "miracle" of saving her daughter.

Years later, after training as a cardiologist and intensivist, I had the opportunity and challenge to transform the lives of thousands of daybetic people in four Latin American countries, both in consultation and in the care of critically ill patients, who struggle between life and death.

From that moment on, helping daybetic people regain their life and health became my Life Mission.

I could share many more stories, but there is one I want you to never forget: not one of my patients treated with my methods died from Covid-19.

Today I can proudly say that my knowledge and the trust placed in me by those who applied my methods changed the sad statistics of this terrible epidemic.

Every day thousands of people with this disease die, and the worst part is that, as has been proven in various scientific studies, most of these deaths are potentially AVOIDABLE.

It is a proven fact that thousands of people with diabetes become regular patients in hospitals, and complications follow one after another.

Their lives no longer belong to them; they have become "hostages of their disease," and pain and suffering separate them, more and more each day, from a full and happy life.

What I am going to tell you now may seem counterproductive, but I want you to know that diabetes mellitus is not an enemy; on the contrary, it is a powerful friend that, understood correctly, helps you find your Life Mission, and it is your responsibility to understand and embrace the changes you need to make in your life with love and resilience.

#iamfreeofcomplications

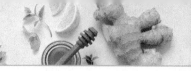

Nothing justifies putting your life at risk; you have the power to make the right choices and start living a full and unlimited life.

The good news is that acute and chronic complications of diabetes mellitus can become fears of the past. If you master what I reveal in this simple yet powerful book, you will learn how to reverse symptoms, reduce medication doses, and be free of complications.

By becoming your own therapist, you will learn how to escape danger and regain confidence and self-control.

After reading this book and applying my methods, the responsibility for your health is in your hands. Make good use of the knowledge I am sharing with you, and let's go on this journey smiling at life.

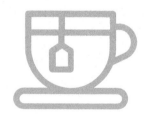

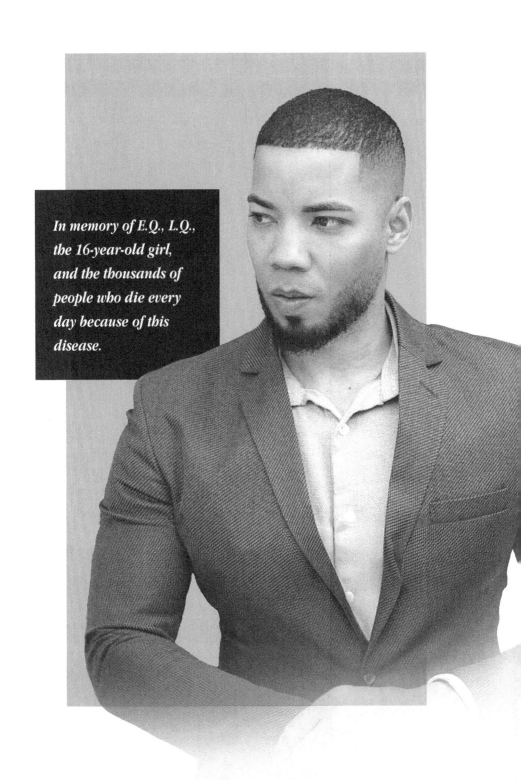

In memory of E.Q., L.Q., the 16-year-old girl, and the thousands of people who die every day because of this disease.

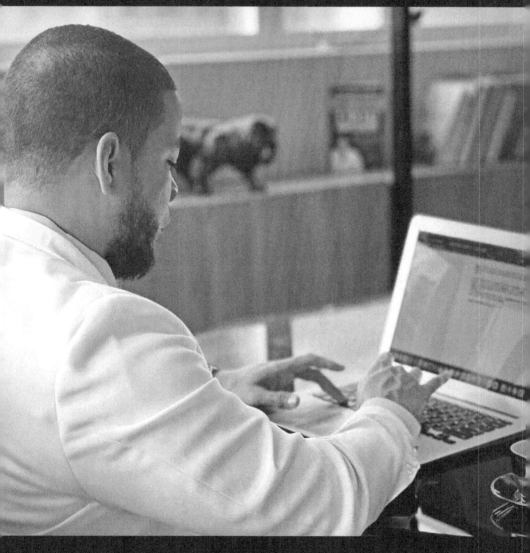

the *end* of
DIABETES
MELLITUS

ESSENTIAL
CON
CEPTS

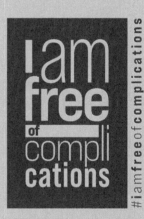

i am
free
of
compli
cations

#iamfreeofcomplications

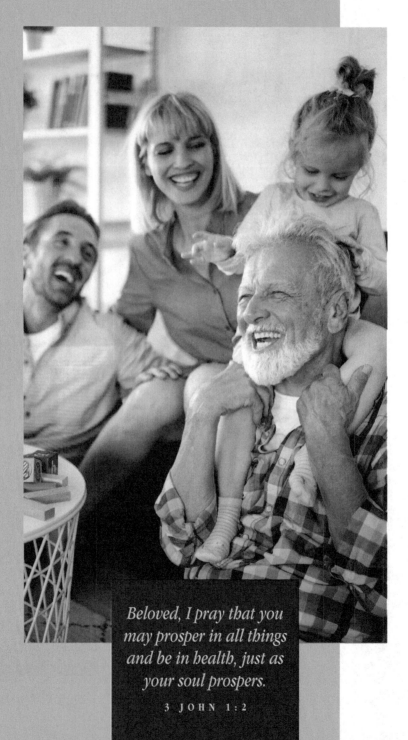

Beloved, I pray that you
may prosper in all things
and be in health, just as
your soul prospers.

3 JOHN 1:2

Diabetes
MELLITUS

D iabetes mellitus, often simply called "diabetes," is a chronic condition that occurs when the pancreas does not produce enough insulin (deficit) or when the body's cells do not respond properly to insulin present in the blood (resistance), resulting in elevated blood sugar (glucose) levels.

A common effect of uncontrolled diabetes is hyperglycemia—elevated blood sugar—which over time can seriously damage various organs and systems in the body, especially nerves and blood vessels, increasing the risk of heart attacks, strokes, acute and chronic kidney diseases, leg ulcers with the risk of amputation, vision loss among other complications.

Identified as an epidemic of the 21st century, in 2020, it was estimated that 9.3% of adults between the ages of 20 and 79, approximately 463 million people, were living with diabetes, and the annual deaths due to preventable causes exceeded 6.7 million people worldwide.

DM ranks 9th among diseases that cause the most loss of healthy life years.

#iamfreeofcomplications

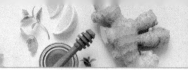

CLASSIFICATION OF DIABETES MELLITUS

TYPES OF DIABETES	
1	**DM type 1:** – **Type 1A:** Insulin deficiency due to autoimmune destruction of the pancreas cells, verified by laboratory tests; – **Type 1B:** Idiopathic cause insulin deficiency.
2	**Type 2 DM:** Progressive loss of insulin secretion combined with insulin resistance.
3	**Gestational DM:** Hyperglycemia of varying degrees daygnosed during pregnancy, without previous DM criteria.
4	**Other types of DM:** Monogenic syndromes (MODY). Neonatal diabetes. Secondary to endocrinopathies. Secondary to diseases of the exocrine pancreas. Secondary to infections. Secondary to drug consumption.
*DM: Diabetes Mellitus; MODY: Maturity-Onset Diabetes of the Young. Adapted from the American Diabetes Association, 2020.	

TYPE 1 DIABETES MELLITUS

Type 1 Diabetes Mellitus (T1DM) is more common in children and adolescents and is characterized by severe insulin deficiency secondary to the grave destruction of the beta (ß) cells of the pancreas, generally due to autoimmune causes**.

The clinical presentation is characterized by a tendency to develop acute complications such as Ketoacidosis*** and Coma****, which requires insulin therapy from the moment of daygnosis.

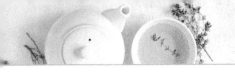
Frequent symptoms at the time of daygnosis:

- Frequent urination (polyuria).
- Constant hunger (polyphagia).
- Excessive thirst (polydipsia).
- Weight loss or lack of weight gain.
- Weakness.
- Fatigue.
- Nausea.
- Vomiting.
- Nervousness.
- Mood changes.
- Loss of consciousness.

 ## *Author's note*

*Hyperglycemia: occurs when the level of glucose in the blood is elevated, above the values established as normal. The main cause of this increase in blood glucose is diabetes.

**Autoimmune Diseases: occur when the immune system does not function correctly and attacks the body's own structures, instead of defending against foreign or dangerous elements, such as viruses, bacteria, and parasites. For reasons that are generally not identified, our immune system "confuses" the body's cells as invading agents and begins to destroy them.

In the case of T1DM, the immune system attacks the body's own healthy cells, specifically the Beta (ß) cells of the pancreas responsible for producing insulin, developing large amounts of autoantibodies against these cells.

***Daybetic Ketoacidosis: is a complication that arises directly from hyperglycemia, i.e., the excessively high concentration of glucose in the blood and low inside the cells, which causes the formation of harmful substances called ketone bodies.

****Coma: is a condition in which there is a reduction or loss of consciousness level, the person appears to be asleep, does not respond to environmental stimuli, and does not show self-awareness.

#iamfreeofcomplications

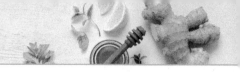

TYPE 2 DIABETES MELLITUS

Type 2 Diabetes Mellitus (T2DM), previously known as non-insulin-dependent diabetes with adult onset, results from a lack of insulin (partial deficiency in insulin secretion by the pancreas' beta cells) and/or insulin's inability to adequately exert its effects (Insulin Resistance*).

It manifests as permanently elevated blood glucose levels - hyperglycemia and may be accompanied by alterations in the secretion of other hormones.

It is the most common type of diabetes, with more than 95% of people with diabetes having this type, largely due to risk factors such as:

- Parents, siblings, or close relatives with diabetes.
- Obesity or overweight.
- Pre-diabetes.
- Having been daygnosed with gestational diabetes or having had a baby weighing over 4 kg.
- Physical inactivity.
- Inadequate lifestyle (smoking, alcoholism, etc.).
- High blood pressure.
- Elevated cholesterol and triglycerides (the latter with a higher risk).
- Use of glucocorticoid class medications**.
- Other risk factors.

 *Insulin Resistance

Occurs when the cells of the muscles, fat, and liver do not respond correctly to insulin and cannot easily absorb glucose from the blood. As a result, the pancreas produces more insulin to help transport glucose into the cells.

Insulin Resistance is generally caused by a combination of genetic influences, inadequate lifestyle, and the presence of diseases such as obesity, high blood pressure, high cholesterol, and triglycerides, among others.

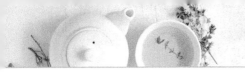

 **Glucocorticoids

Also known as corticosteroids or corticoids, are potent medications derived from the hormone cortisol, which is produced in the adrenal gland.

There are several synthetic formulations of corticosteroids, the most used are Prednisone, Prednisolone, Hydrocortisone, Dexamethasone, and Methylprednisolone.

Initial signs and symptoms

Symptoms can be similar to those of type 1 diabetes mellitus but are generally less intense, so the disease may be daygnosed several years after the first symptoms when complications have already appeared.

Hyperglycemia only causes symptoms when the glucose concentration is very high, generally when it is above 180 to 200 milligrams per deciliter (mg/dl) or 10 to 11.1 millimoles per liter (mmol/l).

Symptoms of hyperglycemia develop slowly over several days, weeks, months, or years. The higher the blood glucose levels, the more severe the symptoms can be. However, some people with type 2 diabetes do not show symptoms for years, despite having elevated blood glucose levels.

Recognizing the symptoms of hyperglycemia quickly can help control and reverse the damage caused by the disease immedaytely, preventing the onset of complications.

#iamfreeofcomplications

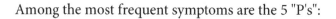

Among the most frequent symptoms are the 5 "P's":

- Polyuria (increased urine volume and frequency).
- Polyphagia (excessive hunger).
- Polydipsia (excessive thirst).
- Unexplained weight loss.
- Pruritus (itching).

Other common symptoms include:

- Fatigue.
- Blurred vision.
- Headache.
- Wounds that are slow to heal.

Evolutionary Signs and Symptoms

If hyperglycemia is not treated, several acute complications can occur. The signs and symptoms that reveal the possible presence of an acute complication are:

- Bad breath.
- Nausea and vomiting.
- Shortness of breath.
- Dry mouth.
- Weak pulse.
- Disorientation.
- Abdominal pain.
- Chest pain.
- Paralysis of a part of the body and/or face.
- Decreased level of consciousness that can lead to coma.

DAYGNOSIS OF TYPE 2 DIABETES MELLITUS

There are various laboratory methods to daygnose diabetes mellitus, and the goal is always to determine the glucose levels in the plasma, which is a component of the blood. It is important that these tests are carried out in specialized and certified facilities for laboratory tests.

We have 4 fundamental tests for daygnosis*:

1. Fasting Plasma Glucose Test (FPG).

2. Oral Glucose Tolerance Test (OGTT).

3. Random Plasma Glucose Test.

4. Glycated Hemoglobin Test - or A1c (HbA1c).

   *Adapted from the American Diabetes Association, 2020.

Fasting Plasma Glucose Test (FPG)

It is the most used for daygnosing diabetes because it is easy to apply and has a low cost.

This test measures the levels of glucose in the blood while fasting. It is important to make sure you are fasting, meaning not having eaten or drunk anything except water, for at least 8 hours before the test.

This exam is performed in the morning, before breakfast.

Importance: to detect the presence of diabetes or prediabetes.

#iamfreeofcomplications

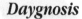

Daygnosis

- **Normal:** less than 100 mg/dl.
- **Prediabetes:** glucose levels between 100 mg/dl and 125 mg/dl (suggests the person is more likely to develop type 2 diabetes mellitus).
- **Confirmed Diabetes:** glucose levels equal to or higher than 126 mg/dl, confirmed by repeating the test on another day.

Oral Glucose Tolerance Test (OGTT)

This type of test measures blood glucose at two moments:

1. After at least 8 hours of fasting.

2. After 2 hours of ingesting a liquid containing a known amount of glucose (75 grams).

Importance: to detect diabetes or prediabetes.

Daygnosis

- **Normal:** less than 140 mg/dl.

- **Prediabetes (also known as glucose intolerance):** glucose levels between 140 mg/dl and 199 mg/dl. This means you are at a higher risk of developing type 2 diabetes.

- **Confirmed Diabetes:** glucose levels equal to or higher than 200 mg/dl, confirmed by repeating the exam on another day.

Random Plasma Glucose Test

In this test, blood glucose is analyzed without considering the time since the last meal, meaning it is performed at any time of the day.

Importance: used to detect diabetes but not prediabetes.

Daygnosis

Random glucose levels equal to or higher than 200 mg/dl in the presence of one or more symptoms (see diabetes symptoms) confirm the presence of diabetes.

Glycated Hemoglobin Test - or A1c (HbA1c)

Doctors may use the HbA1c test alone, or in combination with other exams, to make a daygnosis. This test should be performed in certified laboratories and fasting is not required for its performance.

Importance: indicated to detect the presence of diabetes mellitus and to know the average blood glucose level during the last 90 days prior to the blood draw.

Daygnosis

- **Normal:** less than 5.7%
- **Prediabetes:** 5.7% to 6.4%
- **Confirmed Diabetes:** 6.5% or more

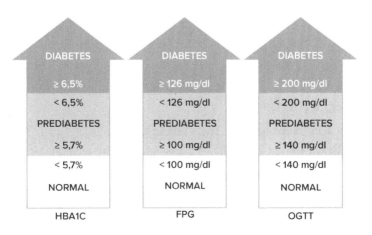

DIABETES	DIABETES	DIABETES
≥ 6,5%	≥ 126 mg/dl	≥ 200 mg/dl
< 6,5%	< 126 mg/dl	< 200 mg/dl
PREDIABETES	PREDIABETES	PREDIABETES
≥ 5,7%	≥ 100 mg/dl	≥ 140 mg/dl
< 5,7%	< 100 mg/dl	< 140 mg/dl
NORMAL	NORMAL	NORMAL
HBA1C	FPG	OGTT

* Adapted from the American Diabetes Association, 2020.

#iamfreeofcomplications

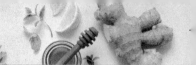

SUMMARY

Classification according to glycemia values

Daygnosis	Fasting Plasma Glucose Test (mg/dl)	Oral Glucose Tolerance Test (mg/dl)	Random Plasma Glucose Test (mg/dl)	Glycated Hemoglobin Test (%)
Normal	<100	<140	N/A	<5.7
Prediabetes	100 to 125	140 to 199	N/A	5.7 to 6.4
Confirmed Diabetes	≥126	≥200	200 with symptoms of hyperg- lycemia	>6.4

Adapted from the American Diabetes Association, 2020.

According to the previous table, the daygnostic criteria for diabetes (ADA, 2020) are as follows:

- **Fasting Plasma Glucose Test:** ≥ 126 mg/dL (after no caloric intake for at least 8 hours).
- **2-Hour Plasma Glucose:** ≥ 200 mg/dL during an Oral Glucose Tolerance Test.
- **Glycated Hemoglobin Test (HbA1c):** ≥ 6.5%.
- **Random Plasma Glucose Test:** ≥ 200 mg/dL with classic symptoms of hyperglycemia.

Causes of Decompensation (Hyperglycemia Peaks)

Among the most frequent are:

- Consumption of foods with a high Glycemic Index.
- Consumption of high-protein foods.
- Increase in the formation of Free Radicals and Advanced Glycation End-products (AGEs).
- Stress and anxiety for any reason.
- Using expired insulin or inadequate doses.
- Consumption of certain medications such as steroids.
- Presence of an infection (blood, teeth, abscess, etc.).
- Not taking hypoglycemic medications (or taking incorrect doses).
- Decompensation of the failure of an organ (heart, kidneys, liver, among others).

COMPLICATIONS OF DIABETES MELLITUS

DM complications are divided into two (2) groups:

- Acute
- Chronic

Acute complications (occur within minutes or hours and can be fatal):

- Hypoglycemia*.
- Ketoacidosis.
- Hyperosmolar coma.
- Acute renal failure.
- Stroke.
- Acute amaurosis (blindness).
- Acute myocardayl infarction.
- Death.

#iamfreeofcomplications

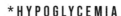

*HYPOGLYCEMIA

Means low blood glucose concentration, a form of sugar in the blood. The human body needs glucose for energy and to carry out the processes necessary to sustain life.

Symptoms include:

- Feeling of hunger.
- Trembling.
- Dizziness.
- Confusion.
- Difficulty speaking.
- Feeling of anxiety or weakness.

In people with diabetes, hypoglycemia is often a side effect of diabetes medications or not eating at the indicated times.

The Natural Therapies proposed in this book will help you control blood sugar as they activate the body's elimination mechanisms, recovering the integrity of the organs most affected by diabetes mellitus such as the brain, the heart, and the kidneys.

Chronic Complications (Long-Term)

Keeping the levels of glucose and other toxic substances such as Free Radicals, Advanced Glycation End-products, and Ammonia in the blood within a healthy range can help prevent chronic complications related to diabetes.

The prolonged maintenance of high levels of glucose and other toxic substances can injure blood vessels, causing them to narrow and thus limiting blood flow to organs.

Once the blood vessels and nerves throughout the body are affected, you can develop various complications associated with diabetes.

Several organs can be affected, particularly the following:

- **Brain:** causing memory loss, Alzheimer's disease, and vascular dementia.

- **Nerves:** causing daybetic neuropathy, which is more common in the lower extremities, and comes with decreased sensitivity in the feet, cramps, pain, ulcers, necrosis, and amputations.

- **Eyes:** glaucoma, cataracts, and daybetic retinopathy, which can lead to vision loss and even blindness.

- **Heart:** high blood pressure and chronic ischemic heart disease.

- **Kidneys:** recurrent infections, daybetic nephropathy which can lead to chronic kidney disease.

- **Immune system:** people with diabetes mellitus are particularly susceptible to bacterial and fungal infections.

- **Reproductive system:** impotence and erectile dysfunction, recurrent infections.

- **Osteoarticular system:** osteoporosis, arthritis, and osteoarthritis.

I'll see you in the next chapter to continue discovering together how to overcome diabetes mellitus.

#iamfreeofcomplications

CONTROL

Workbook

Therapist, on the next page you will find 7 questions to answer based on the concepts you read in the previous chapter. These questions are not casual; mastering the answers will surely bring you much closer to freeing yourself from symptoms, medications, risks, and complications.

Answer them conscientiously,
A big hug

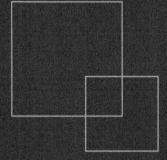

1. The complications of diabetes mellitus are divided into two major groups, acute and chronic:
- ( ) True
- ( ) False

2. If acute hyperglycemia is not treated, acute complications of diabetes mellitus can occur.
- ( ) True
- ( ) False

3. In Brazil, more than 130,000 people die each year due to acute and generally preventable complications of diabetes mellitus.
- ( ) True
- ( ) False

4. Diabetes mellitus affects various organs and body structures such as the brain, eyes, heart, and kidneys.
- ( ) True
- ( ) False

5. In the end, what decides whether a daybetic person will have complications is:
- ( ) The genetic load you have from your parents
- ( ) Their lifestyle

6. Eating foods rich in carbohydrates (High Glycemic Index) is not one of the causes of glucose decompensation in the blood:
- ( ) True
- ( ) False

#iamfreeofcomplications

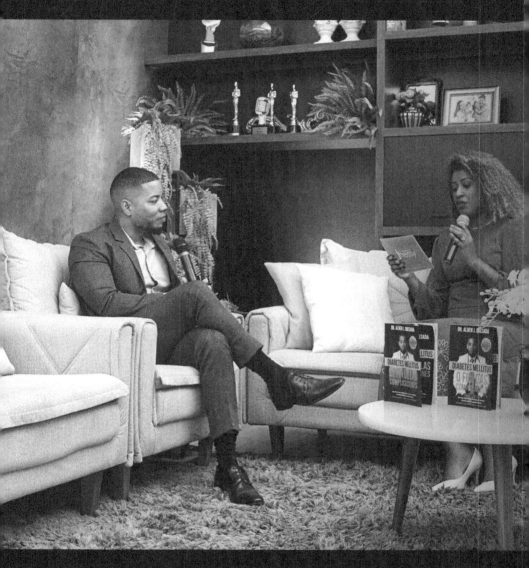

the end of
DIABETES
MELLITUS

NATURAL THERAPIES IN THE TREATMENT OF
DIABETES MELLITUS

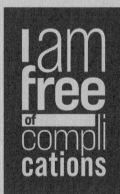

#iamfreeofcomplications

@draldenquesada.es

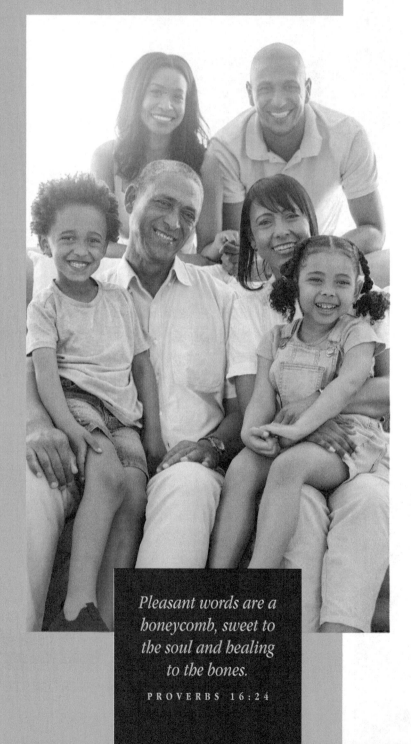

*Pleasant words are a
honeycomb, sweet to
the soul and healing
to the bones.*

PROVERBS 16:24

N atural therapies are those that utilize resources available in nature, or methods that do not harm the organism, to promote health, heal, and prevent diseases.

According to the WHO, the terms "complementary medicine," "alternative medicine," or "natural medicine," refer to a wide range of healthcare practices that are not part of the tradition or conventional medicine of a given country, nor are they fully integrated into the predominant health system.

Natural therapies are used according to the patient's daygnosis, and their goal is always to accelerate the recovery process and reversal of diseases; however, sometimes, their function may be merely palliative.

Traditional Chinese Medicine (TCM) practices include therapeutic procedures and health treatments such as herbal-based medications, acupuncture, and manual therapies like acupressure, chiropractic, osteopathy, and other similar techniques, including qi gong, tai chi, yoga, thermal medicine, and other physical, mental, spiritual, and psychophysical therapies.

I was introduced to the world of natural therapies through my father, who was a doctor recognized in his state as an orthodox physician, but he realized that by prescribing pharmaceutical industry medications, he could not reverse the damage of diseases. On the contrary, he saw how his patients worsened year after year, as was the case with my two daybetic cousins.

He, my father, began to apply various natural therapies with excellent results, and I remember that the lines of people in despair at his clinic were endless.

#iamfreeofcomplications

My calling for natural therapies emerged when I saw how people who had lost all hope regained their health after receiving the natural treatments he applied.

After completing my training as a doctor and cardiologist, I decided it was time to honor my father's legacy and began to study his treatment protocols again.

I discovered incredible things; he had noted the progression of many of his patients, which were literally his scientific studies where he recorded the evolution of symptoms, medications, among other clinical and pharmacological-therapeutic variables, something wonderful.

100% of his patients improved satisfactorily with his naturalist treatment protocols.

I began to study and delve deeper into natural therapies, to better understand the functioning of the body as a whole rather than in fragments as we are taught in medical school.

I also had an advantage; I had trained as a scientific researcher and had access to hundreds of clinical trials on the beneficial effects of plants and other natural therapies, published in prestigious medical libraries like Pubmed.

That's how I created my own therapeutic system, unifying and harmonizing conventional-orthodox medicine with natural therapies that were studied in large clinical trials and where their efficacy was demonstrated.

In other words, instead of treating body alterations with medications, which do not reverse cell damage, etc., I created a system, combining and harmonizing various natural therapies, that can stimulate the

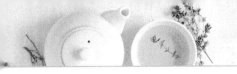
process of eliminating toxic substances from the body and reverse, to a large extent, the damage caused by diseases.

The big difference between what most therapists apply and the proposal of this book is that many of them, without belittling their work for a second, apply one or at most three techniques, which undoubtedly is beneficial for the human body, but it is not enough to stimulate the healing process in all its dimensions.

For illustrative purposes, it's unlikely that a professional who applies acupuncture and acupressure will be able to help their daybetic patients, as they are not addressing the main challenge of a person with this disease: nutrition.

On the other hand, a specialist in natural therapies who masters Macrobiotics, Phytotherapy, and Fruit Therapy- among other therapies that stimulate the body's detoxification process- can help people with chronic diseases, especially those directly related to nutrition, to reverse the damage- understand the symptoms and most of the complications- caused by these.

And precisely this was one of the greatest contributions I made with my research.

I discovered how to combine the most powerful natural therapies, those with scientific studies proving their effectiveness, in a harmonious way that accelerates the reversal of cell damage, Biological Age, and Body Detoxification.

In summary: when we combine some simple, but powerful natural therapies, and apply them at specific times of the day, which correspond with human body cycles, we stimulate the process of reversing cell, tissue, and organ damage, in a 100% effective way.

#iamfreeofcomplications

After treating thousands of daybetic people around the world and meticulously studying the evolution of each of them, I was able to identify their bodies' responses to the method and what objectives we could achieve throughout the Body Detoxification process.

Natural History of Damage Reversal

This concept, created by me, is based on the results I have had with my patients, where 100% of them managed to eliminate symptoms and reverse neurological, renal, and cardiovascular damage in 30 days.

According to my research conducted with my patients, the objectives achieved with naturopathic treatment can be divided into two main groups:

- General objectives
- Time-based (evolutionary) objectives

General objectives

- Detoxify the body.
- Reverse Biological Age*.
- Control glycemia.
- Reverse symptoms.
- Reduce or eliminate medication dosages.
- Eliminate the risk of developing acute and chronic DM complications.
- Control all blood parameters and cardiovascular risk factors.

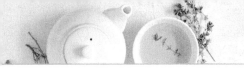 *Biological Age

Biological Age is a measure of an individual's physiological functioning and health in relation to their chronological age, that is, their actual age in years. This includes the state of the cells, organs, and the efficiency of the processes that keep us alive.

Biological Age is like your body's internal clock that measures how much time has passed since you were born in terms of how your body is functioning.

Although we all have a real age in years, our internal parts, such as bones, muscles, and organs, also age, and some do so faster than others, as in the case of daybetics.

For example, a person with diabetes mellitus who is 45 years old, their organs may be 55 years old in Biological Age or more if other diseases and alterations such as obesity, hypertension, hypercholesterolemia, hypertriglyceridemia, etc., are present.

It's the famous phrase: "I may look fine on the outside, but I'm destroyed on the inside..."

The good news is that by performing the body detoxification protocol proposed in this book, it is possible to reverse the Biological Age and match it to the Chronological Age, thus reversing the damage caused by the disease.

#iamfreeofcomplications

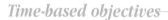

Time-based objectives

If you commit to 100% of the method for 30 days, this is what you can expect:

From 0 to 3 days applying the method

1. Absolute control of glycemia, avoiding acute complications.

2. The intensity of symptoms begins to decrease.

3. Reduction of Physical and Psychological Hunger.

4. You start to sleep better without the need for medication.

From 3 to 7 days applying the method

1. Absolute control of glycemia, avoiding acute complications.

2. You begin to reduce the dosages of normoglycemic medications (fast and slow insulin, metformin, gliclazide, etc.).

3. Almost complete reversal of symptoms such as: leg pain and cramps, fatigue and lack of energy, discouragement, lack of sexual appetite, among others.

4. Psychological Hunger continues to decrease.

5. Insomnia disappears.

It is important to highlight that when symptoms begin to decrease, it is because the neurological, renal, and cardiovascular damage is being reversed, that is, the body is undergoing the process of repair and regeneration of all its structures at the cellular, tissue, and organ levels.

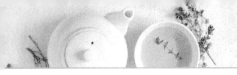

From 7 to 28 days applying the method

1. Absolute control of glycemia, avoiding acute and chronic complications.

2. Complete reversal of symptoms, healing of ulcers, improvement of vision, libido, and sexual performance.

3. Control of blood pressure and blood parameters (cholesterol, triglycerides, renal function, etc.).

4. The need for the use of normoglycemic medications (fast and slow insulin, metformin, gliclazide, etc.) continues to decrease until it is finally possible to eliminate them all or maintain minimal dosages.

5. You will lose between 6 kg and 14 kg of body weight in 30 days or regain your ideal weight if you are below your ideal weight.

6. Absolute control of Psychological Hunger.

7. Replenishment of all essential nutrients.

8. Increase in energy and disposition.

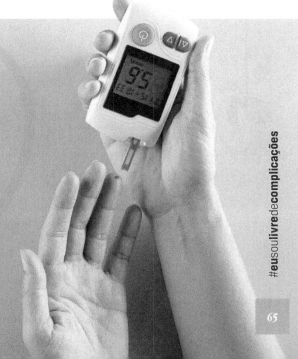

#eusoulivredecomplicações

- Absolute control of glycemia, avoiding acute complications.

- The intensity of symptoms begins to decrease.

- Reduction of Physical and Psychological Hunger.

- You start to sleep better without the need for medication.

- Absolute control of glycemia, avoiding acute complications.

- You begin to reduce the dosages of normoglycemic medications (fast and slow insulin, metformin, gliclazide, etc.).

- Almost complete reversal of symptoms such as: leg pain and cramps, fatigue and lack of energy, discouragement, lack of sexual appetite, among others.

- Psychological Hunger continues to decrease.

- Insomnia disappears.

NATURAL HISTORY OF DAMAGE REVERSAL

- Absolute control of glycemia, avoiding acute and chronic complications.

- Complete reversal of symptoms, healing of ulcers, improvement of vision, libido, and sexual performance.

- Control of blood pressure and blood parameters (cholesterol, triglycerides, renal function, etc.).

- The need for the use of normoglycemic medications (fast and slow insulin, metformin, gliclazide, etc.) continues to decrease until it is finally possible to eliminate them all or maintain minimal dosages.

- You will lose between 6 kg and 14 kg of body weight in 30 days or regain your ideal weight if you are below your ideal weight.

- Absolute control of Psychological Hunger.

- Replenishment of all essential nutrients.

- Increase in energy and disposition.

 Goals by time
Results you will have after starting to use the method.

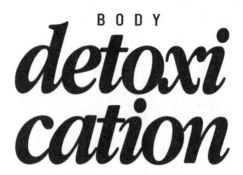

BODY
detoxi cation

Now, I imagine you must be wondering:

Well, how do natural therapies work to achieve these spectacular results?

And the answer is:

Through Body Detoxification, which is a wonderful natural process of eliminating accumulated toxins in the body, responsible for most, if not all, chronic diseases.

The Body Detoxification process is carried out in key organs such as the liver, kidneys, and intestines, which work together to filter and eliminate toxins.

These organs perform a vital task, but sometimes they can be overwhelmed by an excessive toxic load due to our modern lifestyle, which includes unhealthy diets, excessive stress, and exposure to pollutants like medications and environmental contaminants.

This excessive overload of toxins is also responsible for the worsening of diabetes mellitus and the emergence of symptoms and complications.

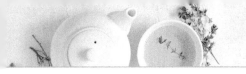
Without going into details, as it is not the aim of this book, it's important for you to know that the body has 4 powerful natural mechanisms for eliminating toxins:

- The skin (through sweat).
- The kidneys (through urine).
- The liver and intestines (through fecal matter).
- The lungs (through oxygenation and CO_2 elimination).

By stimulating these mechanisms in the correct way, at the correct times, and with the correct combinations of natural therapies, we can "force" our body to eliminate in a few days the toxins accumulated over years, which are responsible for the dysfunction of the pancreas and other affected organs, insulin resistance, hyperglycemia, and the need for medication.

A concept that I consider extremely important to remember again, because you must master it, is that of Healthy Eating.

Although we are going to use various natural therapies to reverse the damage caused by DM, Healthy Eating - it is worth remembering - is the fundamental pillar of Body Detoxification.

A Healthy Food must meet 5 principles:

1. During its cultivation and harvesting process, it was not contaminated with pesticides, etc.

2. It is in its natural or minimally handled condition when consumed.

#iamfreeofcomplications

3. The more you eat, up to the point of feeling satisfied, the more beneficial it is for your health as it provides the essential macro and micronutrients for proper cellular function.

4. It can be ingested both in the presence of health and disease, and it does not accelerate the progression of damage; on the contrary, it stimulates the reversal of symptoms.

5. Its consumption, in a rationally adequate amount, does not increase your blood glucose levels because it has a Low or Moderate Glycemic Index and Glycemic Load.

If you carefully read these 5 principles, you'll see how far we are today from having a Healthy Diet.

To better understand what constitutes a Healthy Food (or diet), let me share a very illustrative example with you:

Often, your doctor or endocrinologist may suggest you can have milk with coffee and whole wheat bread with cheese or margarine for breakfast. But what happens after this breakfast?

Generally, your blood sugar levels will increase, and you might think this is "normal," a result of diabetes mellitus, without realizing that this hyperglycemia is secondary to a breakfast completely devoid of Healthy Foods.

The good news is that in the upcoming chapters, you'll learn how to correctly and 100% naturally stimulate the Body Detoxification process to reverse the damage caused by diabetes mellitus.

SYNDROME
detoxification

When someone starts a Body Detoxification process, it's common to experience a range of symptoms in the first few days.

These symptoms are the body's response to the release of toxins and changes in internal chemical balance. The most common symptoms include:

- Headache.
- Nausea and dizziness.
- Weakness.
- Cramps.

- Blurred vision.
- Irritability.
- Skin changes.
- Among others.

These symptoms are due to the body's "reaction" to a process of change and are an excellent sign that your body is undergoing a wonderful detoxification process and eliminating all toxins.

If these symptoms appear, you should not worry; instead, you should proceed as follows:

1. Be thankful, as they reflect that spectacular changes are happening in your body.

2. Lie down for a few minutes and drink the Normoglycemic Tea or Cucumber Juice to stay hydrated.

#iamfreeofcomplications

These symptoms can last up to 7 days, never more than that time, and when they disappear, you will experience an incredible level of energy and readiness.

 Dr. Quesada's Suggestion

If the symptoms persist for more than 7 days, or are very intense, I suggest you consult a doctor as soon as possible.

After this period, which I call the Hyper-toxemia Period because it is due to an excess of toxins in the blood that the body needs to eliminate, my patients often tell me:

"Dr. Quesada, I am electric with so much energy."

Body Detoxification is an important step towards improving health and overall well-being, and soon, the benefits far outweigh the initial symptoms.

In conclusion, Body Detoxification is a fundamental process for freeing the body from accumulated toxins. The initial symptoms can be challenging, but with proper hydration-nutrition and rest, it is possible to quickly and effectively deal with them.

 Important note

If these symptoms do not appear, you should not worry either because it is due to two fundamental facts:

- Either your body was not overloaded with toxins.
- Or the 4 mechanisms of bodily elimination are working perfectly well and eliminated the toxins quickly.

We continue to move forward...

My goal is for you to become your Own Therapist.

Workbook

CONTROL

CHAPTER 3

Therapist, on the following page, you have **5 questions** to answer based on the concepts you read in the previous chapter. It's important that you master the objectives of natural therapies to reverse the damage caused by diabetes mellitus..

Answer them conscientiously,
A big hug

1. Carrying out the Body Detox protocol proposed in this book, it is possible to reverse the Biological Age and match it to the Chronological Age, thus we will be able to reverse the damage caused by the disease.

◯ True
◯ False

2. When we combine simple, yet powerful natural therapies, and apply them at specific times of the day, which correspond to the human body's cycles, we stimulate the process of reversing cellular, tissue, and organ damage in a 100% effective way.

◯ True
◯ False

3. When symptoms begin to decrease, it is because the neurological, renal, and cardiovascular damage is being reversed, that is, the body is carrying out the process of repair and regeneration of all its structures at a cellular, tissue, and organ level.

◯ False
◯ True

4. If symptoms associated with Body Detoxification appear, all you have to do is lie down for a few minutes and drink the Normoglycemic Tea or the Cucumber Juice.

◯ False
◯ True

5. All the foods recommended in this book meet the concept of Healthy Eating and have a Low Glycemic Index and Load.

◯ False
◯ True

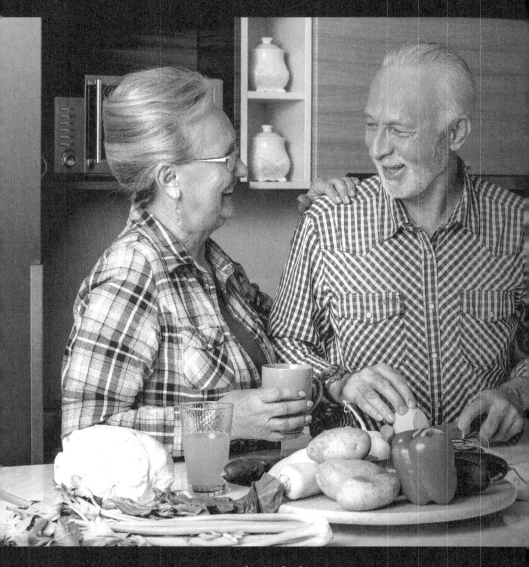

the *end* of
DIABETES
MELLITUS

IMPORTANCE OF HEALTHY EATING IN REVERSING

DIABETES MELLITUS

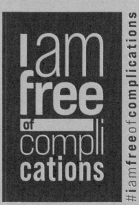

i am free of compli cations

#iamfreeofcomplications

@draldenquesada.es

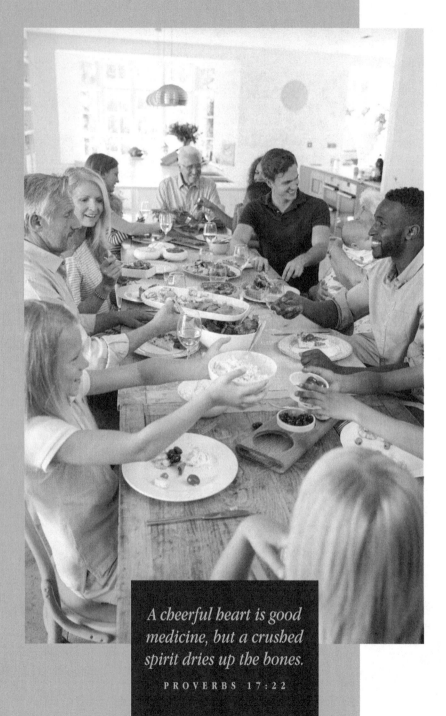

*A cheerful heart is good
medicine, but a crushed
spirit dries up the bones.*

PROVERBS 17:22

Numerous medications and technologies have been developed for the control of diabetes mellitus, but, undoubtedly, one aspect that continues to be an irreplaceable pillar in its treatment is diet.

The food we consume is not merely a source of pleasure or energy; it is essentially the raw material that our body uses to regulate processes that maintain health or generate diseases, especially those acquired and known as chronic.

If we think carefully, every bite of food is a decision we make for or against our health.

When facing DM, diet plays a role not only in the immediate control of blood sugar but also has a profound impact on the prevention of short and long-term complications.

Making healthy daily dietary choices will make a difference between maintaining stable health or facing acute episodes of hypoglycemia or hyperglycemia and complications.

Adhering to a consistent and conscious Healthy Eating regimen will protect us from the appearance of chronic complications, such as heart disease, kidney diseases, or neurological damage like nerve damage.

Now, to better understand how dietary choices affect the control of DM and the prevention of complications, I propose that we address two indicators that help predict the impact of foods on blood sugar response.

#iamfreeofcomplications

These indicators are:

- The Glycemic Index (GI)
- The Glycemic Load (GL)

Glycemic Index

The concept was introduced by Jenkins et al., at the beginning of the last century, as a classification system for carbohydrates (CHOs), based on their immediate impact on glucose levels.

The GI shows how foods containing the same amount of carbohydrates can have different effects on glucose levels.

When ingesting foods with carbohydrates, they are broken down in the body into glucose, our main energy fuel. The process of transformation and the speed at which glucose is released into the blood vary depending on the type of carbohydrate.

While simple carbohydrates can cause sharp spikes in glucose - hyperglycemia - within about 15 minutes, complex carbohydrates, rich in fiber, take between one and two hours to do so, helping to maintain a constant balance in our glucose levels.

Here's a simple explanation of the GI concept:

Imagine that all the carbohydrates you consume are like trains carrying sugar to your blood. The GI tells you how fast that train (carbohydrate) delivers its sugar load to the blood.

It's important to highlight that this system helps us classify carbohydrates into Low, Moderate, or High Glycemic Index, based on their impact on glucose levels.

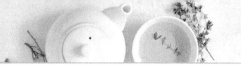
Classification of foods according to the GI

Based on how they raise blood sugar levels when compared to a reference carbohydrate: glucose (GI 100).

1. **Low GI (55 or less):** these foods are digested, absorbed, and metabolized slowly, resulting in a gradual increase in blood glucose. Generally, they take between one and two hours to do so.

2. **Medium GI (56-69):** these foods have an intermediate impact on blood glucose levels.

3. **High GI (70 or more):** these foods break down quickly in the digestive system and release glucose into the blood at a faster rate, usually starting about 15 minutes after ingestion.

Rapid Glycemic Response

Occurs when we eat foods with a High GI. The glucose from these foods is absorbed quickly, causing spikes in hyperglycemia.

This rapid rise in blood sugar triggers a response from the body, releasing a large volume of insulin to deal with this excess sugar. However, this rapid increase in glucose levels is often followed by a sharp drop, which can cause fatigue and an increased sense of hunger.

Some scientific research has found that people who consume diets with a High GI have less satiety, leading to excessive food intake, favoring an increase in body weight and levels of Glycosylated Hemoglobin.

#iamfreeofcomplications

Moreover, consuming foods with a high GI can alter the lipid profile and insulin secretion, favoring the onset of cardiovascular diseases and worsening diabetes mellitus.

The consumption of high GI foods appears to trigger a sequence of hormonal events in the postprandial period, causing more hunger and excessive food intake.

Slow Glycemic Response

Is the result of consuming foods with a Low GI.

These foods release glucose into the bloodstream more gradually, contributing to a slower and steadier rise in blood sugar levels, translating into a more constant and lasting energy release.

An important fact is that eating low GI foods can help prevent spikes and drops in glucose levels, which is particularly important for diabetic individuals.

It has also been proven that low GI foods can help maintain a feeling of fullness for longer, which is beneficial for avoiding Psychological Hunger and weight gain.

Additionally, the intake of low GI foods can decrease the secretion of counter-regulatory proteolytic hormones like cortisol, growth hormone, and glucagon, stimulating protein synthesis.

Some scientific research shows that the regulation of body fat mass associated with the intake of low GI diets may be related to gene activation.

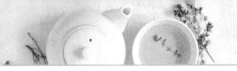
It was observed that the intake of low GI foods tends to increase the content of lean mass and significantly decrease body fat content, favoring the control and reversal of the damage caused by diabetes mellitus.

Factors Affecting Glycemic Index:

- **Variety:** white rice has a higher Glycemic Index than brown rice.

- **Fiber:** the fiber content in a starch can act as a barrier to the action of amylases and slow down absorption. The higher the fiber content, the lower the GI.

- **Cooking:** hydration and heat tend to increase the GI. Avoid overcooking pasta and potatoes until they become too soft.

- **Temperature:** when starch is cooked and then cooled down, its GI decreases. Pasta, rice, or potatoes, when cooled, have a lower GI.

- **Ripeness:** the riper the fruit, the higher its GI. Choose fruits that are ripe but not overripe.

- **Combinations:** in some carbohydrates, the natural content of proteins can cause a slower hydrolyzation of the starch and lower its GI. Include legumes in your diet as they contain proteins in their composition.

- **Presentation:** whole foods or those in pieces are absorbed more slowly than liquids. It is preferable to consume tubers, fruits, and vegetables in pieces or whole, rather than in purees or juices.

It's crucial to highlight that the Glycemic Index is not the only factor to consider when planning a diet, especially for people with diabe-

#iamfreeofcomplications

tes. Other aspects, such as the total amount of carbohydrates, the nutritional quality of foods, and the Glycemic Load (which we will discuss later), are also essential.

Lastly, always remember that it's necessary to have the guidance of a healthcare professional or a nutritionist when making significant changes to your diet based on the GI.

Glycemic Load

The Glycemic Load is a combination of the GI and the amount of carbohydrates (HC) in a food. It is obtained by multiplying the Glycemic Index of the food by the available carbohydrates (in grams) and dividing that result by 100.

GL = GI * amount of HC (g) / 100

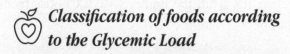 **Classification of foods according to the Glycemic Load**

- **Low Glycemic Load:** 1 to 10
- **Medium Glycemic Load:** 11 to 19
- **High Glycemic Load:** 20 or higher

Recalling the explanation of the train that carries sugar to the blood, the GL refers to how much sugar that train is carrying.

Unlike the Glycemic Index, which only takes into account the quality of the carbohydrates to be consumed, the GL includes the amount of carbohydrates in a serving of food, making it a more advisable method for glucose management.

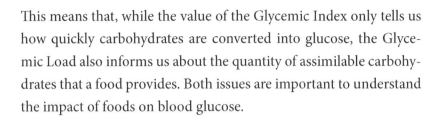

This means that, while the value of the Glycemic Index only tells us how quickly carbohydrates are converted into glucose, the Glycemic Load also informs us about the quantity of assimilable carbohydrates that a food provides. Both issues are important to understand the impact of foods on blood glucose.

The GL tells us about the intensity of the insulin response that a food we are going to consume will provoke because a food can have a high GI, but if it has few carbohydrates, its GL could be low.

When we talk about assimilable, or available, carbohydrates, we are referring only to those that will produce an increase in glucose. Fiber, despite being part of carbohydrates, is not absorbed, so it is not taken into account for calculating the Glycemic Load.

Therefore, all foods that a diabetic person should consume, if they wish to reverse the damage caused by this disease and avoid complications, must comply with 5 fundamental principles to be a Healthy Food:

1. Was not contaminated with pesticides, etc., during its cultivation and harvesting process.

2. Is in its natural state or minimally processed at the time of consumption.

3. The more you eat until you feel satisfied, the more beneficial it is for your health because it provides the essential macro and micronutrients for proper cellular function.

4. Can be consumed both in the presence of health and in the presence of diseases, and does not accelerate the progression of damage; on the contrary, it stimulates the reversal of symptoms.

#iamfreeofcomplications

5. Its consumption, in a rationally adequate amount, does not increase your blood sugar levels because it has a Low or Moderate Glycemic Index and Load.

Therefore, all foods that a diabetic person should consume, if they aim to reverse the damages caused by this disease and avoid complications, must meet these 5 fundamental principles.

You might think it's challenging to adapt to the concept of Healthy Eating, but never forget that the rewards are immense if you invest in yourself, your future, and your well-being.

Every food choice is an opportunity to strengthen your health, to provide your body with the "fuel" it needs to function optimally.

It's time to reflect and ask ourselves:

Am I making the right food choices for my well-being?

Is what I do daily worsening my disease, or am I building health, freedom, and happiness?

Honest answers to these questions will undoubtedly make you a better person...

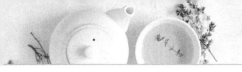
✎ *Important note*

All foods recommended in this book comply with the concept of Healthy Food and have a low Glycemic Index and Load.

Foods to Avoid

Lastly, to complete our understanding of what constitutes Healthy Eating, there are a group of foods recognized as detrimental to health or may not be the best for aiding the process of reversing the damage caused by diabetes mellitus.

These foods should always be avoided, or at least for the 30 days you are undergoing your Body Detoxification process.

By excluding these foods from your meals, you will be supporting:

- The body's detoxification process.
- Blood glucose control.
- Reversal of biological age, symptoms, and diseases.

Avoid consuming:

1. **Milk and its derivatives:** cheese, ice cream, flavored yogurt, etc.

2. **Fats:** margarine, butter, refined oils, etc.

3. **Foods with chemical additives:** colorants, preservatives, flavorings, cube seasonings, etc.

4. **Foods processed through genetic engineering techniques:** refined flours, chocolate, coffee, fried foods, pickles (preserved), smoked foods, sodas, white sugar, candies.

#iamfreeofcomplications

5. **Animal-derived foods:** red meats (pork and beef), processed meats (bologna, chorizo, salami, ham, etc.), and seafood like shrimp, crabs, and lobsters.

6. **Refined flour:** sweets, cakes, bread, etc.

7. **Beverages:** alcohol and its derivatives (beer, rum, etc.), carbonated and processed drinks (including all those sold in boxes as "natural", as they contain preservatives).

 Important note

- When you go shopping, take the Food List proposed at the end of this book and be consistent; resist the temptation to buy any of the foods to avoid or those not on the Shopping List.
- If you have any of these foods to avoid at home, and it's feasible, consider donating them to someone you know who is not ill. Do so with great joy, feeling happy that you are in control of your decisions and choosing to be a person free from symptoms and complications.

Regarding the Consumption of Animal Proteins

You are advised not to eat any type of meat, especially red meat, during the 30 days of Body Detoxification.

The end product of the meat we ingest, in addition to amiño acids, is ammonia.

Ammonia is an extremely toxic gas that needs to be converted into uric acid so it can be eliminated by your kidneys.

Diabetes mellitus affects your kidneys, and if you are someone who consumes a lot of animal proteins, it's likely your kidneys are overloaded with toxins and have some degree of damage. Therefore, we will limit their consumption to improve this situation and enhance kidney function.

The proteins recommended in this guide for 30 days are of plant origin, are of high biological value, and have excellent properties for regenerating cells, tissues, and organs damaged by DM.

To make it easier to understand the power of adhering to a diet where the main source of protein is plant-based, here is an example:

Most of my patients with some degree of renal insufficiency see improvement in all clinical and laboratory parameters (creatinine, uric acid, glomerular filtration, etc.) after eliminating meats, especially "red" meats, for 30 days.

Plant-Based Protein Sources Recommended in This Protocol:

- Chickpeas
- Lentils
- Beans
- Quinoa
- Miso
- Among others

#iamfreeofcomplications

Important Notes

1. The desire to eat animal meat may feel "uncontrollable" and might cause you a bit of anxiety. If this happens, don't worry; include a small portion of chicken or fish cooked in a pressure cooker with water, salt, onion, garlic, rosemary, and other natural spices once a day, especially at lunch, and only combine it with the indicated vegetables. Gradually decrease the frequency of meat consumption until it's just twice a week.

2. Never combine meats with potatoes, sweet potatoes, taro, yams, cassava, or any other carbohydrate source, as your blood glucose will spike rapidly after consuming these foods.

CHAPTER

Notes

CONTROL

Workbook

Therapist, on the following page you will find **5 questions** based on the concepts you read in the previous chapter. It's crucial that you understand the significance of nutrition in reversing the damage caused by diabetes mellitus and that you grasp some basic concepts that will aid you on your journey.

Answer them thoughtfully,
Warm regards

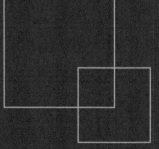

1. To reverse the damage caused by diabetes mellitus, healthy eating is generally more important than medication, especially in the early stages of the disease.

○ True
○ False

2. When facing DM, Healthy Eating not only plays a significant role in the immediate control of glycemia but also has a profound impact on preventing complications in the short, medium, and long term.

○ True
○ False

3. Choosing healthy foods daily will make the difference between maintaining good health or experiencing acute episodes of hypoglycemia or hyperglycemia and complications.

○ False
○ True

4. Simple carbohydrates can cause sharp spikes in glucose - hyperglycemia - within approximately 15 minutes. Complex carbohydrates, rich in fiber, take between 1 and 2 hours to do so, contributing to more stable glycemia levels.

○ False
○ True

5. All foods recommended in this book meet the Healthy Eating concept and have a Low Glycemic Index and Glycemic Load.

○ False
○ True

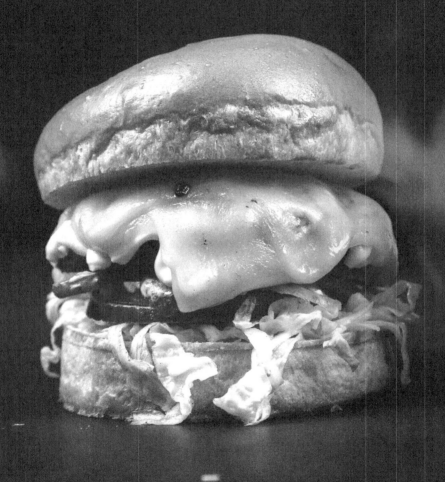

the end of
**DIABETES
MELLITUS**

FOOD COMPULSION AND

DIABETES MELLITUS

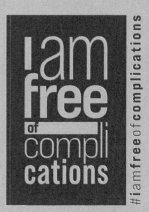

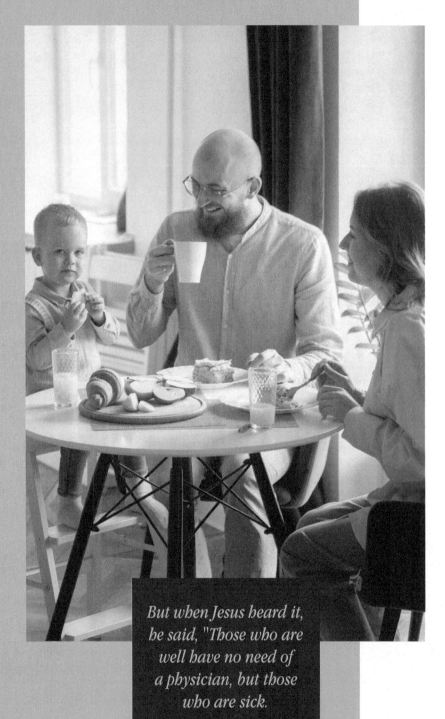

the end of
**DIABETES
MELLITUS**

*But when Jesus heard it,
he said, "Those who are
well have no need of
a physician, but those
who are sick.*

MATTHEW 9:12

I n the complexity of human beings, food transcends the mere function of subsistence and intertwines with our emotional, cultural, and psychological fabric.

We live in an era where food is more accessible than ever, yet paradoxically, we also face an alarming increase in food-related disorders.

Anxiety and Food Compulsion (FC), in particular, have emerged as a silent but significant challenge, affecting individuals across all strata and ages of our society.

The relationship each individual has with food is unique, and this relationship can reflect how we relate to ourselves and the world around us.

While some find refuge and comfort in food, others may feel trapped in a cycle of overeating followed by guilt and self-reproach.

Despite these individual variations, one thing is certain: eating goes beyond simply satisfying hunger.

If you've ever wondered, "Why am I eating if I'm not hungry?" or "Why do I turn to food when I feel anxious, overwhelmed, or sad?", you're not alone.

These are fundamental questions we'll address in this chapter, shedding light on the distinction between Physical Hunger and Emotional Hunger, and we'll discover tools to overcome Emotional Hunger and balance our relationship with food.

As we proceed on this journey, I invite you to open your mind and heart, to approach this issue not as a battle to be won, but as an opportunity for self-discovery and personal growth.

#iamfreeofcomplications

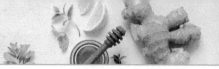

Addressing Food Compulsion is not just about weight or body shape but about how we choose to live and relate to ourselves and others.

Food Compulsion

As seen in the previous chapter, food is a fundamental pillar in the onset of diabetes mellitus and in the disease's negative as well as positive progression.

Our relationship with food is multifaceted and, in many cases, complex. Like any other human behavior, eating can be influenced by a multitude of internal and external factors.

In this context, it's crucial to understand a phenomenon that has gained prominence in the discussion on health and wellbeing: Food Compulsion.

Food Compulsion (FC) can be described as an uncontrollable urge to eat, often in large amounts and without feeling real hunger.

This action is not carried out for the pleasure of tasting or enjoying food but is rather an impulsive act, an attempt to fill a void that is not necessarily physical.

It's as if the person is being swept away by an underlying current, where the act of eating becomes an automatic response to certain stimuli or emotional states.

It's important to understand that everyone, at some point, may experience episodes of overeating. Perhaps after a particularly exhausting day, or during a family celebration.

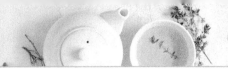

However, the difference lies in the frequency and motivations behind the act.

While occasional overeating is a shared experience by many, FC is a recurring behavior, often linked to specific emotions or situations.

Individuals experiencing Food Compulsion often describe feelings of loss of control during episodes, followed by guilt, shame, and remorse.

The concern is that these feelings can fuel the cycle, creating a spiral where compulsive eating becomes a habitual way of coping with emotions and stress.

Finally, it's crucial to differentiate Food Compulsion from other eating disorders, like Bulimia Nervosa.

Although both involve episodes of excessive intake, in Bulimia, these episodes are followed by purgative behaviors, such as self-induced vomiting or excessive use of laxatives.

Now, let's get to know two fundamental concepts:

- Physical Hunger and Emotional Hunger

Physical Hunger vs. Emotional Hunger

Our body and mind operate in an impressive synergy. Both have ways of communicating with us, and understanding these messages is essential for cultivating a healthy relationship with food.

Two of the most prevalent, and often confused, signals we experience are Physical Hunger and Emotional Hunger.

#iamfreeofcomplications

Physical Hunger

This is our body's biological demand for energy. It is a natural and necessary process for survival.

Manifestations:

- It presents gradually and can wait.
- The stomach sends signals like growling or a feeling of emptiness.
- There may be symptoms like weakness, lack of concentration, or irritability.
- Generally, a prolonged period of time, more than 3 hours, has passed since the last food intake.
- You don't have a preference for any specific type of food; you need to eat.
- Satisfaction after eating: consuming food and satisfying Physical Hunger, you experience a feeling of fullness and satiety.
- There are no negative feelings associated with having eaten.

Emotional Hunger (Psychological)

This is where food becomes a response not to a physical need but to an emotional state.

Manifestations:

- It appears suddenly in response to emotions, such as stress, sadness, boredom, or even happiness.
- There are no physical signs that the body needs food.
- Usually, a short period of time has passed since the last food intake.
- It's not linked to the need for energy but to a desire for comfort or relief. In this case, you're not feeding the body but an emotional need. Food acts as a distraction or as a form of self-reward.
- You crave specific foods like pizza, a hamburger, ice cream, etc.

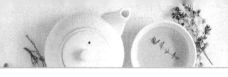

- Lack of satiety: despite consuming large amounts of food, you may not feel satiated or fulfilled, as the origin of the "hunger" is not physical.

- After eating, you feel guilty and emotionally punish yourself.

Factors Contributing to Food Compulsion

Like many human behaviors, CA does not arise from a single isolated factor; it is the result of a combination of internal and external influences that interact and can intensify the tendency to eat compulsively. Understanding these influences is crucial to addressing the issue from its root and creating effective strategies to manage it.

Without going into detail, as it is not the focus of this book, I share some of the factors that contribute to the emergence and perpetuation of CA:

- Psychological Factors
- Social and Cultural Pressures
- Traumatic Experiences
- Hormonal Imbalance
- Extreme Dietary Restriction
- Body Image Issues
- Environmental Factors

Psychological Factors

Anxiety, stress, boredom, loneliness, sadness, or frustration can trigger episodes of compulsion. Food becomes a tool to manage these emotions, albeit durationrarily.

#iamfreeofcomplications

In the fight against Food Compulsion, awareness is a powerful tool. Recognizing and understanding the factors contributing to this behavior is an essential step toward recovery and developing a healthier, more balanced relationship with food.

Social and Cultural Pressures

Beauty Standards: We live in a society that idolizes a certain body type, which can generate pressure to conform to those standards. This pressure can trigger unhealthy eating behaviors.

The Culture of "Comfort Food": Food is often promoted as a solution for emotional well-being: "chocolate for heartbreak," "ice cream for sad days," etc.

Traumatic Experiences

People who have experienced traumas, whether in childhood or adulthood, may turn to food as a form of self-comfort or to suppress painful memories.

Hormonal Imbalance

Hormones play a crucial role in regulating appetite and satiety. Hormonal imbalances, such as altered levels of leptin or ghrelin, can influence hunger and satiety patterns.

Extreme Dietary Restriction

Adopting strict or restrictive diets can lead to episodes of overeating. The body may react to food deprivation by storing energy when the opportunity arises.

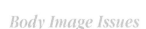

Body Image Issues

Dissatisfaction with one's body can lead to cycles of extreme diets followed by episodes of overeating, especially if the person feels frustrated with their weight loss progress.

Environmental Factors

Being constantly surrounded by food, living in an "obesogenic environment" where processed and unhealthy food is easily accessible, can increase opportunities and temptations to eat compulsively.

This analysis of contributing factors is a key piece in the puzzle of Food Compulsion. Identifying and understanding these factors can provide a solid foundation for developing intervention and prevention strategies.

Consequences of Food Compulsion

- Physical Consequences
- Psychological and Emotional Consequences
- Social Consequences

The impact of CA extends beyond occasional excessive intake. It affects both the body and the mind, generating consequences that can be both short and long-term. Understanding these consequences is crucial when addressing and managing this issue.

#iamfreeofcomplications

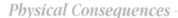

Physical Consequences

- **Weight Gain:** recurrent intake of large amounts of food, especially those high in calories, can lead to weight gain which, over time, can lead to obesity.

- **Digestive Problems:** compulsive episodes can cause stomach discomfort, indigestion, acid reflux, or constipation.

- **Chronic Diseases:** food Compulsion can increase the risk of diet and weight-related diseases, such as type 2 diabetes, heart diseases, and certain types of cancer.

- **Hormonal Imbalances:** food Compulsion can disrupt hormones related to appetite and satiety.

Psychological and Emotional Consequences

- **Guilt and Shame:** after an episode, it's common to feel guilty or ashamed, which can further fuel the compulsion cycle.

- **Low Self-Esteem:** the perceived lack of control during and after episodes can negatively affect personal image and self-worth.

- **Depression and Anxiety:** there is a bidirectional relationship between Food Compulsion and these conditions; compulsion can be both a cause and a consequence.

- **Social Isolation:** individuals may avoid social situations for fear of judgment or due to the shame associated with their behavior.

Social Consequences

- **Relationship Difficulties:** tensions and misunderstandings related to eating can arise among friends, family, or partners.

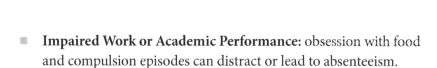
- **Impaired Work or Academic Performance:** obsession with food and compulsion episodes can distract or lead to absenteeism.

- **Financial Problems:** purchasing large amounts of food for compulsive episodes can lead to financial issues.

The consequences of Food Compulsion are multifaceted and can infiltrate nearly all aspects of a person's life. Recognizing and understanding these consequences is a crucial step towards devising strategies to address the problem.

The good news is that with the right support and tools, overcoming Food Compulsion and building a healthy relationship with food is possible.

Therapeutic Tools to Overcome Food Compulsion

After understanding the essential concepts about Food Compulsion, I will reveal the most powerful techniques to conquer this situation which, as we've seen, might be affecting your quality of life.

It's important to know that there are 3 essential moments related to eating and Food Compulsion:

- Before eating
- During the act of eating
- After finishing eating

Mastering and practicing some therapies and exercises for each of these moments, with the aim of reprogramming your mind, I assure you that in a few days you'll be free from this alteration and in full control of your emotions and actions.

#iamfreeofcomplications

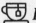 ## Recommendations to Perform Before Meals

1. No Pact.
2. Shopping List.
3. Recommendations for Controlling Anxiety:
   - Deep breathing.
   - Positive visualization.
   - Conscious decision (Think before eating).
4. Normoglycemic Tea.

No Pact

To change your daily habits, you must commit to saying No to all situations and behaviors that you know distance you from your goal of controlling and reversing the damage of DM.

The No Pact works as an "Internal Guardian", as we usually operate on autopilot, meaning we perform actions without thinking, eating, and drinking more than necessary, then feeling guilty afterward.

So, write in a notebook the No Pact:

"I (your name) commit to saying No to everything that harms me. From now on, I will only do what's best for my health and will not fall victim to temptation.

I have the power to decide about my life and refuse to be prey to impulses, no matter how tempting they may be. I embrace myself because I am the most incredible human being that exists and deserve to live my life in health and happiness."

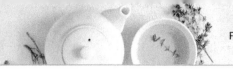
 Dr. Quesada's Suggestion

I suggest repeating this Pact out loud several times a day.

Shopping List

In chapter 9, you have a powerful Food List for detoxifying the body.

Whenever you go shopping, take the list with you and commit to only buying what's indicated. This way, you'll be controlling the impulse to buy harmful foods that affect your health.

Deep Breathing

Take a few minutes for some deep breaths.

Close your eyes, inhale slowly counting to four, hold your breath for a second, and exhale counting to four.

This technique helps to calm the nervous system and center the mind, preparing you for conscious eating.

Positive Visualization

Imagine how you feel after eating a moderate dish. Visualize yourself satisfied, energized, and proud of your choices.

Conscious Decision (Think Before Eating)

Ask yourself: Do I have Physical Hunger or Emotional Hunger?

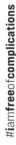

#iamfreeofcomplications

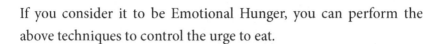

If you consider it to be Emotional Hunger, you can perform the above techniques to control the urge to eat.

Normoglycemic Tea before Meals

Remember that you have indicated Tea 30 minutes before main meals. This will help decrease the sensation of hunger.

Recommendations to Perform While Eating

1. Place and remove food from the plate.
2. Keep food away from the table.
3. Eat slowly.
4. Mindful eating (presence).
5. Pause halfway through the meal.
6. Chew 20 times each bite until reaching 50 times.
7. Finish the dish of food in no less than 10 minutes.
8. Talk with fellow diners between bites.
9. Get up from the table after finishing your plate of food.

Place and Remove Food from the Plate

Serve yourself food on the plate, then remove some of the food you've served. This way, you're controlling your impulse to eat more than necessary.

Keep Food Away from the Table

If possible, request not to place the pots of food on the table, including dessert. This helps avoid the urge to serve yourself again after you've finished your plate of food.

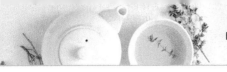

Eat Slowly

Take the necessary time to thoroughly chew each bite. This allows the signals of satiety to reach your brain, helping you recognize when you're full.

Mindful Eating

Concentrate on the flavors, textures, and aromas of your food. Turn off distractions like the TV or phone and avoid eating standing up or in a rush.

Pause Mid-Meal

When you've eaten half of your plate, take a pause and assess your level of hunger and satiety. Consciously decide whether to continue eating or if you're already satisfied.

Chew 20 Times Each Bite up to 50 Times

This is an excellent technique for controlling anxiety as people often eat too quickly and don't chew their food properly, delaying the satiety signal to the brain.

Finish the Dish of Food in No Less Than 10 Minutes

Take the time to chew each bite thoroughly. This allows the signals of satiety to reach your brain and helps you recognize when you're full.

Talk with Fellow Diners Between Bites.

Establish a family atmosphere free of problems and worries, remember the exercises of Presence, I Am Here, and I Am Now.

#iamfreeofcomplications

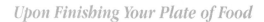

Upon Finishing Your Plate of Food

The moment you finish your plate of food, get up from the table; don't wait to eat dessert.

If you struggle with self-control, talk to your family members and explain that you need their help to not "fall into temptation"; please serve dessert after you have finished and are no longer at the table.

Recommendations for After Eating

1. Emotional Journaling.
2. Digestive Walk.
3. Gratitude and Self-Acknowledgment.
4. Foot Bath - Breathing Exercise.

Emotional Journaling

Write down how you feel after eating. Are you satisfied, full, still hungry? Recording your emotions can help you recognize patterns and adjust your habits for the future.

Digestive Walk

If possible, consider taking a short walk. It not only aids digestion but also serves as a way to separate the act of eating from returning to daily activities, avoiding snacking on additional food after eating.

Gratitude and Self-Acknowledgment

Take a moment to express gratitude for the meal you've just consumed and positively acknowledge your efforts to eat mindfully. Self-affirmation can strengthen your healthy habits in the long term.

Foot Bath - Breathing Exercise

Every day, upon waking, perform the foot bath for 30 minutes in the mornings and at 9:00 pm. While doing the foot bath, listen to the Relaxation Audio and practice the Breathing Exercise.

✎ Important Notes

1. These techniques complement each other, and it's not necessary to apply them all. You can test one by one and then do the ones that give you the best results.

2. Food Compulsion is not a sign of weakness or lack of willpower. It is a complex response to a variety of factors that can be addressed and managed with the right knowledge and support.

3. In the case of diabetes mellitus, it's crucial to know how to control the sometimes excessive urge to eat without feeling hungry and, above all, to consume sweets and foods known to be harmful.

#iamfreeofcomplications

CONTROL

Workbook

CHAPTER 5

Therapist, below are **5 questions** for you to answer based on the concepts you read in the previous chapter. Food Compulsion and Psychological Hunger are "disorders" that we must pay special attention to avoid falling into the trap of compulsively eating foods that accelerate the onset of neurological, renal, and cardiovascular damage...

Answer them conscientiously,
A big hug

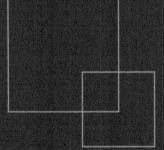

1. Food Compulsion can be described as an uncontrollable desire to eat, often in large quantities, without feeling real hunger.
- ( ) True
- ( ) False

2. People who experience Food Compulsion generally describe feelings of loss of control during episodes, followed by guilt, shame, and remorse.
- ( ) True
- ( ) False

3. In Emotional Hunger (psychological), food becomes a response not to a physical need, but to an emotional state.
- ( ) False
- ( ) True

4. It's not important to have a Shopping List when going to the market, as you can buy whatever you want, regardless of the quality of the food.
- ( ) False
- ( ) True

5. In the Pact of No to change your daily habits, you must commit to saying No to all situations and behaviors that you know will take you away from your goal of controlling diabetes.
- ( ) False
- ( ) True

CHAPTER 6

GENERAL
RECOM
MENDA
TIONS

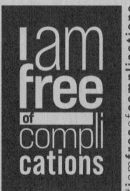

i am
free
of
compli
cations

#iamfreeofcomplications

@draldenquesada.es

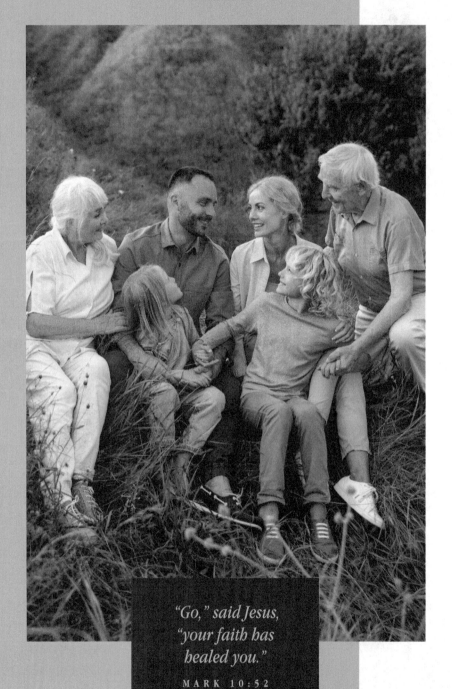

the end of
DIABETES
MELLITUS

*"Go," said Jesus,
"your faith has
healed you."*

MARK 10:52

D ear Therapist, below I share with you everything you need to reverse the damage caused by diabetes mellitus and be free from symptoms, medications, risks, and complications.

As you will see, these are general, simple, yet very powerful recommendations that will make a difference in your life, impacting your health, finances, and, not least, family stability.

What you need to apply the method:

1. Discipline and perseverance.

2. A device to monitor blood glucose -glucometer-.

3. Purchase some natural foods and products.

4. A thermos (500ml or 1 liter) and thick straws.

5. A small bowl in case you need to take lunch to work.

6. A basin for the Footbath.

7. Headphones to listen to the Mental Reprogramming audios, Breathing and Relaxation exercises.

#iamfreeofcomplications

Dr. Quesada's Advice

If you have an Alexa device - or similar - or the possibility to buy one, you can configure daily indications by setting alarms, reminders, and the Mental Reprogramming, Relaxation, and Breathing Exercises audios.

Such a device will be very useful, especially for the indications you have before getting out of bed and before sleeping.

Where to Start

As I mentioned before, and I would like to reinforce, you should apply the method for 30 continuous days. I know it will be a challenge for you, and that is why I have structured all the indications so that they are easy to understand and, above all, easy to apply.

In the following chapter, which is the most important of this book, you will see the indications by time of day, and I would like you to start by taking the first step, which would be, from my point of view, to read the book and buy the foods listed in the Shopping List.

It is worth remembering that in the final chapter of the book, you will find how to prepare the Recipes and the Shopping List.

My suggestion is that starting tomorrow, you begin preparing the Normoglycemic Tea and Cucumber Juice, as these are very powerful, economical, and easy-to-make indications that will bring immediate benefits.

I also invite you to consider having a family meeting and sharing that you are starting a new journey in your life, so all support to meet your goals is welcome.

I am sure you will receive help to make your transformation smoother and more harmonious.

I urge you to study and master all the indications you have for your day, so you can know what you are doing right and what you could improve on.

Finally, I want you to be aware of your progress, to have control and mastery over what you are doing every day, so you can accompany your transformation and recover your state of health-freedom.

I'll see you in the next chapter because you are one step away from becoming your Own Therapist!

#iamfreeofcomplications

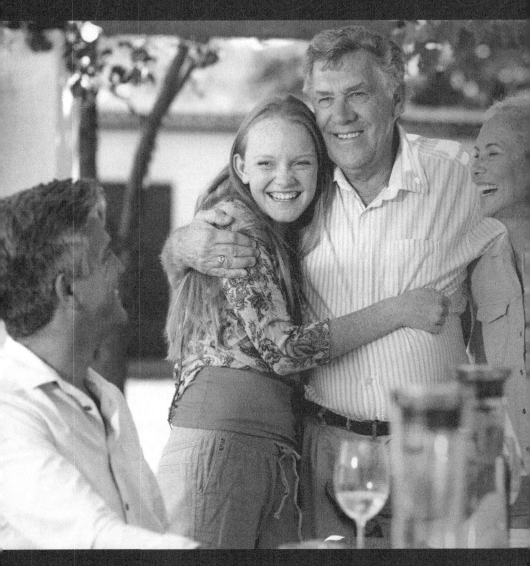

the end of
DIABETES
MELLITUS

CHAPTER 7

DAILY RECOM MENDA TIONS

TO REVERSE THE DAMAGE OF DIABETES MELLITUS

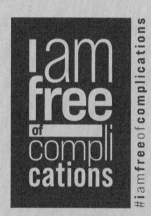

i am free of compli cations

#iamfreeofcomplications

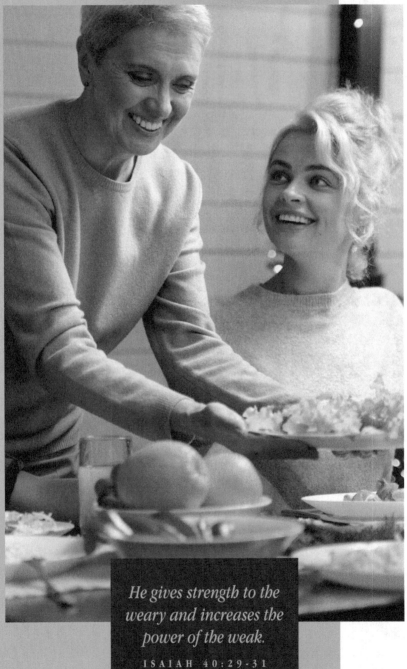

the end of
DIABETES MELLITUS

> *He gives strength to the weary and increases the power of the weak.*
>
> ISAIAH 40:29-31

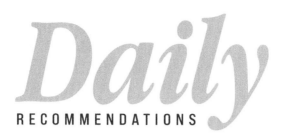

Daily

RECOMMENDATIONS

D ear therapist, in the following pages, you will find recommendations, organized by specific schedules and instructions, that you must follow every day to reverse the neurological, renal, and cardiovascular damage caused by diabetes mellitus.

These instructions are based on various scientific studies that have proven their effectiveness and, above all, that they are free from adverse effects.

As you will notice, for lunch, you have indicated 5 different types of Brown Rice recipes and 5 Detoxifying Soup recipes for dinner.

To emphasize:

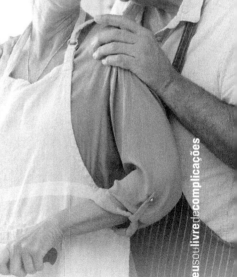

- For lunch, you should only eat one Brown Rice recipe of your preference, accompanied by a raw or steamed vegetable salad.

- For dinner, you should only eat one Detoxifying Soup recipe of your preference, accompanied by a raw or steamed vegetable salad.

#eusoulivredecomplicações

To make it easier for you, and as a mere guideline, I propose 5 lunch and dinner menus - from Monday to Friday - but feel free to make any combination of Brown Rice and Detoxifying Soup any day of the week.

The rest of the instructions remain the same for 30 days.

It's also important to remember that in the upcoming chapters, you will find all the information on how to make and prepare the recommendations.

 Important Notes

1. Respect the schedules, but if it's difficult for you to follow the recommended timing, I suggest you look for options. In other words, you can perform the recommendations before or after the indicated time, but do not skip them.

2. You should never prepare lunch recipes for dinner or vice versa.

3. If you work outside your home, I suggest carrying the Normoglycemic Tea, Cucumber Juice, and Lunch in thermoses.

4. It's crucial to always have your doctor's oversight, especially if you have any pre-existing health conditions.

Lastly, in addition to the Daily Recommendations, you will have 3 Control Tables.

- The first table is for tracking your blood glucose levels at specific times of the day and monitoring your progress.

- The second table is for marking off the daily therapeutic recommendations as completed.

- The third table is for monitoring the evolution of your symptoms.

These three Control Systems work together to provide an effective monitoring of the diabetes mellitus damage reversal after starting the Body Detoxification program.

Measuring blood glucose at specific times, keeping track of daily recommendations, and monitoring symptom evolution help keep the process under strict control, reducing the risk of severe complications and failures in the program.

It's vital that you commit to recording the requested information daily, giving you the confidence and assurance needed to take one more step towards your freedom every day.

 Dr. Quesada's Advice

Strive to follow the program as indicated, sticking to the recipes and proposed schedules with discipline and commitment.

#iamfreeofcomplications

Upon waking up
before getting out of bed

Listen to the Mental Reprogramming audio

Perform Postural Correction and Hypopressive exercises

7:00 am - 7:30 am
Fasting

8:00 am - 8:30 am
Breakfast

10:00 am - 10:30 am
Morning Snack

Upon standing

Conduct the first blood glucose check

2 hours after Breakfast

Conduct the second blood glucose check

MORNING INSTRUCTIONS

10 minutes before lunch
Immune-Boosting Shot

12:00 pm - 1:00 pm
Lunch

4:00 pm - 4:30 pm
Afternoon Snack

10 minutes before Dinner
Immune-Boosting Shot

7:00 pm - 8:00 pm
Dinner

9:00 pm - 9:30 pm
Normoglycemic Tea
Pediluvium

10:00 pm - 10:30 pm
Detoxifying Shot

3

2 hours after
Lunch

Conduct the
third blood
glucose check

4

2 hours after
Dinner

Conduct the
fourth blood
glucose check

AFTERNOON-EVENING INSTRUCTIONS

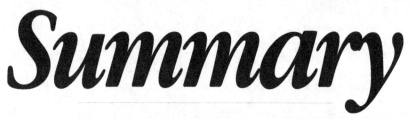

Summary

OF DAILY RECOMMENDATIONS

UPON WAKING UP - *before getting out of bed*

1. Listen to the Mental Reprogramming audio.

2. Perform Postural Correction and Hypopressive exercises.

7:00 AM - 7:30 AM - *fasting*

Start your day by:

1. Drinking Normoglycemic Tea accompanied by Garlic and Aloe Vera.

2. Doing the Pediluvium with Breathing Exercises.

8:00 AM - 8:30 AM - *breakfast*

I propose 3 excellent options:

- Natural Cherry Juice with Ginger and Turmeric
- Natural Orange Juice with Ginger and Turmeric
- Natural Pineapple Juice with Ginger and Turmeric

Important note: You can drink two large glasses of one of the options until you feel satisfied, as they are potent anti-inflammatory juices.

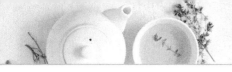
10:00 AM - 10:30 AM - *morning snack*

Prepare Cucumber Juice with Bitter Melon, Cherry, Chayote, and Lemon.

> **Important note:** You can drink two large glasses of this juice until you feel satisfied, as it is a potent normoglycemic juice.

12:00 PM – 1:00 PM - *lunch*

1. **10 minutes before lunch:**
   Immune-Boosting Shot

2. **I propose 5 excellent options:**
   - Brown Rice with Chickpeas
   - Brown Rice with Quinoa
   - Brown Rice with Corn
   - Brown Rice with Lentils
   - Brown Rice with Millet or Barley

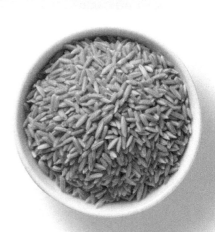

Important Notes

1. Always accompany the Brown Rice recipes with plenty of raw or steamed Vegetables Salad, dressed with Lemon, Sea Salt, and Apple Cider Vinegar.

2. Don't forget to add Linseed, Chia, and Sesame - Sesame Seed- (powdered is better) on top of your meals, after being served at the table.

4:00 PM - 4:30 PM - *afternoon snack*

Prepare and drink Cucumber Juice with Bitter Melon, Cherry, Chayote, and Lemon.

> **Important note:** You can drink two large glasses of this juice until you feel satisfied, as it is a potent normoglycemic juice.

#iamfreeofcomplications

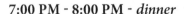

7:00 PM - 8:00 PM - *dinner*

1. **10 minutes before Dinner:** Immune-Boosting Shot

2. **I propose 5 excellent options:**
   - Barley Stew
   - Lentil Soup
   - Corn Soup
   - Miso Soup
   - Millet and Sweet Vegetables Soup

 Important Notes

1. Always accompany the Soup recipes with plenty of raw or steamed Vegetables Salad, dressed with Lemon, Sea Salt, and Apple Cider Vinegar.

2. Don't forget to add Linseed, Chia, and Sesame - Sesame Seed- (powdered is better) on top of your meals, after being served at the table.

9:00 PM - 9:30 PM - *normoglycemic tea - pediluvium*

1. Prepare the Normoglycemic Tea from Rosemary, Cinnamon, Bauhinia forficata, and Guava leaf, adding the juice of a Lemon when it's warm enough to drink.

2. Prepare the Pediluvium, and as you do it, enjoy your delicious Normoglycemic Tea while listening to Relaxing Music accompanied by Breathing Exercises.

10:00 PM - 10:30 PM - *Detoxifying Shot*

After having the Normoglycemic Tea and doing the Pediluvium, it's recommended to prepare a shot of Extra Virgin Olive Oil with the juice of one (1) Lemon.

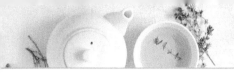
✎ *Important note*

This Shot might be unpleasant to the palate, so I suggest you take it in one gulp, without "thinking twice", or add a pinch of Honey, provided that it's confirmed the ingestion of Honey does not increase your blood sugar levels.

In the following pages, you will find the description of the Instructions by specific times, their goals, and important notes to ensure the success of your process to reverse the damage caused by diabetes mellitus. Let's do this together!

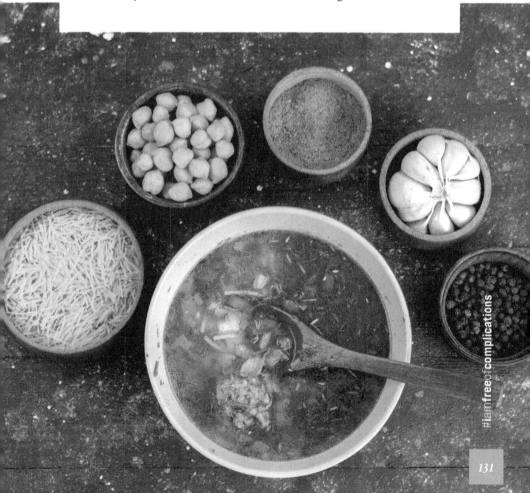

#iamfreeofcomplications

upon waking up

BEFORE GETTING OUT UPON OF BED

- Mental Reprogramming Audio
- Hypopressive Exercises

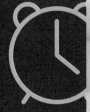

RECOMMENDED TIME
Upon waking up, after opening your
eyes and before getting out of bed.

DURATION: 3-5 minutes
(1 minute for each exercise).

☆ *Objectives*

- Create a positive mental attitude.
- Increase energy and disposition.
- Control food compulsion.
- Eliminate fluid retention.
- Reduce abdominal circumference.
- Stimulate intestinal functioning.
- Promote the body's elimination process of toxic substances.

♡ *Recommendation*

Upon waking, as soon as you open your eyes, the first thing I recommend you do is:

- Listen to a Mental Reprogramming audio.
- Perform 3 Postural Correction and Hypopressive exercises:
  1. Knees to chest
  2. Hip rotation
  3. Hip lift

✎ *Important Notes*

1. This indication is the first thing you should do in the day, i.e., if you wake up at 10:00 am, it's the first thing you should do.

2. If you have a sound device like Alexa, you can set an alarm to wake up with the Mental Reprogramming Audio, otherwise, you can search for the audios on YouTube, Spotify, etc.

3. The three exercises should be performed in bed, and the step-by-step description of how to do them is in the Recipes and Procedures chapter.

4. In case you have contraindications for doing postural exercises, simply skip them, just listen to the Mental Reprogramming audio.

#iamfreeofcomplications

133

fasting

- Normoglycemic Tea
- Foot Bath
- Breathing Exercises

🎯 Objectives

- Control blood sugar levels.
- Reduce Physical and Psychological Hunger.
- Strengthen immunity.
- Promote the body's natural toxin elimination process.
- Stimulate the regeneration process and reverse the damage of the body's cells, tissues, and organs.

RECOMMENDED TIME

7:00 am - 7:30 am

♡ Recommendation

Upon waking up, prepare the Normoglycemic Tea with Rosemary, Cinnamon, Cow's Foot, and Guava leaves, adding the juice of one Lemon when ready to drink and it has cooled to a warm temperature.

While waiting for the Normoglycemic Tea to cool down, prepare the Foot Bath (Chapter 10).

Once the Foot Bath is ready, immerse your feet in the water for 30 minutes and start drinking the Normoglycemic Tea.

Accompany the tea with 2 pieces of previously frozen Aloe Vera and one (1) clove of Garlic, finely chopped just before consuming.

Take a sip of tea and, between sips, perform 2 deep abdominal breaths looking towards the Sun, until you finish the entire cup.

While performing the Foot Bath, you can play some relaxing music to start the day in harmony.

Important Notes

1. If you are allergic to any ingredient, simply do not consume it. Prepare the tea with the other indicated ingredients.

2. This is the first action you should take after waking up, e.g., if you wake up at 10:00 am, this should be the first thing you do.

3. Prepare 1 ½ liters of this Normoglycemic Tea and drink it as regular water at the recommended times.

- **07:00 am** Have a cup on an empty stomach.
- **11:30 am** Have a cup 30 minutes before Lunch.
- **02:00 pm** Have a cup 2 hours after Lunch.
- **06:30 pm** Have a cup 30 minutes before Dinner.
- **09:00 pm** Have a cup 2 hours after Dinner.

4. If you have a fluid intake restriction due to a condition such as Heart or Renal Failure, only prepare the amount of Normoglycemic Tea as recommended by your doctor.

5. Do not add any sweetener - sugar or similar - to sweeten the Tea.

6. Never add Lemon juice to hot beverages, as it loses its beneficial properties.

 Regarding Aloe Vera

1. If you have any degree, or suspicion, of Renal Failure, do not consume Aloe Vera.

2. If you have no contraindications, consume Aloe Vera for 30 days, then rest for 30 days, and repeat the cycle (10 days of consumption - 30 days without taking it).

#iamfreeofcomplications

135

breakfast

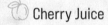 Cherry Juice   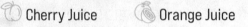 Orange Juice   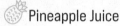 Pineapple Juice

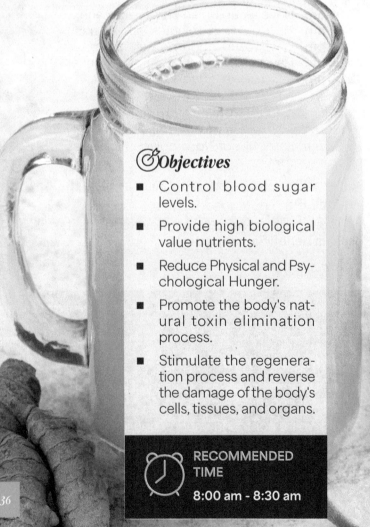

Objectives

- Control blood sugar levels.
- Provide high biological value nutrients.
- Reduce Physical and Psychological Hunger.
- Promote the body's natural toxin elimination process.
- Stimulate the regeneration process and reverse the damage of the body's cells, tissues, and organs.

RECOMMENDED TIME
8:00 am - 8:30 am

Recommendation

After completing the fasting recommendations, I suggest waiting about 1 hour before
consuming Breakfast. This enhances the proper absorption of Aloe Vera and Garlic.

I propose 3 excellent options:

- Natural Cherry Juice with Ginger and
  Turmeric.

- Natural Orange Juice with Ginger and
  Turmeric.

- Natural Pineapple Juice with Ginger and
  Turmeric.

You can have two large glasses of one of these
options, until you feel satisfied, as they are potent anti-inflammatory juices.

Important Notes

1. If you are allergic to any ingredient, simply
   do not consume it. Prepare the juice with
   the other indicated ingredients.

2. This is the first food intake you should
   have in the day, always after the fasting
   recommendation.

3. Do not add any sweetener - sugar or similar - to sweeten the recipes.

4. The amount of Ginger and Turmeric should
   be to taste, pleasant to the palate.

#iamfreeofcomplications

MORNING
snack

Cucumber Juice with Cundeamor, Cherry, Chayote, and Lemon

🎯 *Objectives*

- Control blood sugar levels.
- Control blood pressure.
- Strengthen immunity.
- Provide nutrients of high biological value.
- Reduce Physical and Psychological Hunger.
- Promote the body's natural toxin elimination process.
- Stimulate the regeneration process and reverse the damage of the body's cells, tissues, and organs.

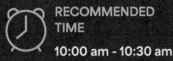

RECOMMENDED TIME

10:00 am - 10:30 am

Recommendation

After completing the recommendations for Fasting and Breakfast, I suggest a very important snack to continue detoxifying the body and providing nutrients.

Proposal

Prepare a Cucumber Juice with Cundeamor, Cherry, Chayote, and Lemon.

You can have two large glasses of this juice, until you feel satisfied, as it is a potent anti-inflammatory and normo-glycemic agent.

Important Notes

1. If you are allergic to any ingredient, simply do not consume it. Prepare the Juice with the other indicated ingredients.

2. It is not mandatory to take this juice in the mornings, especially if you wake up late, as you should prioritize the Fasting and Breakfast recommendations.

3. All ingredients should be "to your taste," without forcing the doses.

4. Do not add any sweetener - sugar or similar - to sweeten.

5. I suggest you drink the juice with a straw, one sip every 30 seconds, so it doesn't become unpleasant.

6. You can prepare a larger quantity of this juice, carry it to work in a thermos, and drink whenever you feel hungry.

7. If you have a daily liquid intake restriction due to a condition such as Heart or Renal Failure, you should prepare the amount of Juice according to your doctor's recommendation.

#iamfreeofcomplications

IMMUNE-BOOSTING

shot

Apple Cider Vinegar and Propolis

 Objectives

- Control blood sugar levels.
- Eliminate free radicals.
- Promote digestion.
- Strengthen immunity.

RECOMMENDED TIME

10 minutes before Lunch and Dinner for 30 days.

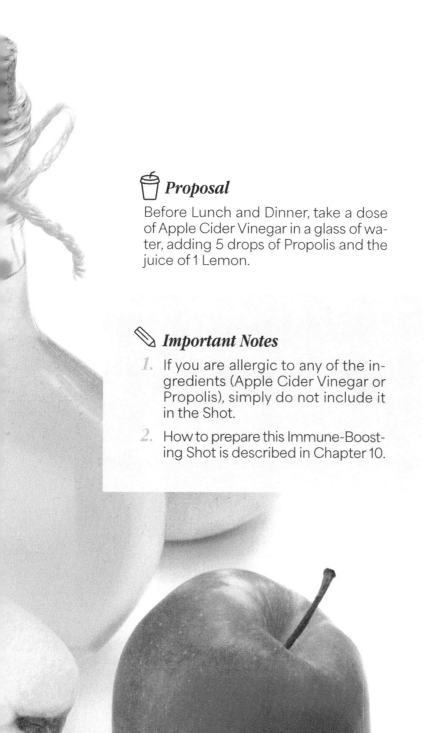

🥤 *Proposal*

Before Lunch and Dinner, take a dose of Apple Cider Vinegar in a glass of water, adding 5 drops of Propolis and the juice of 1 Lemon.

✎ *Important Notes*

1. If you are allergic to any of the ingredients (Apple Cider Vinegar or Propolis), simply do not include it in the Shot.

2. How to prepare this Immune-Boosting Shot is described in Chapter 10.

#iamfreeofcomplications

lunch

BROWN RICE WITH VEGETABLES

⊙ Objectives

- Prevent spikes in blood sugar levels.
- Strengthen immunity.
- Provide nutrients of high biological value.
- Control Physical and Psychological Hunger.
- Stimulate the process of regeneration and reversal of damage to cells, tissues, and organs.

RECOMMENDED TIME

12:00 pm - 1:00 pm

♡ *Recommendation*

1. Prepare and take the Immune-Boosting Shot 10 minutes before Lunch.

2. Lunch marks the start of the solid food intake for the day, making it of great importance. To fulfill the purpose of detoxifying the body, these foods must be rich in nutrients that promote the process of nutrition and cellular repair.

I propose 5 excellent options:

- Brown Rice with Lentils
- Brown Rice with Chickpeas
- Brown Rice with Quinoa
- Brown Rice with Corn
- Brown Rice with Millet or Barley

⟋ *Sugestões*

- You should accompany the Brown Rice recipes with plenty of raw or steamed vegetable salad.

- It is important to sprinkle Flaxseed, Chia, and Sesame (preferably in powder form) over your meals after serving.

✎ *Important Notes*

1. If you are allergic to any ingredient, simply do not use it; prepare the recipes with the other indicated products.

2. This indication is your first solid meal of the day, so you should stick to the suggested recipes so the body receives foods rich in macro and micronutrients of high biological value that promote the process of repair and cellular restoration.

3. You can eat until you feel satisfied, without restriction on quantity, but you should prioritize the intake of vegetable salad.

4. Avoid drinking water or any other liquid during and up to 1 hour after meals.

5. Chew each bite of food between 20 and 50 times until it is completely crushed in your mouth.

#iamfreeofcomplications

AFTERNOON
snack

Cucumber Juice with
Bitter Melon, Cherry,
Chayote, and Lemon.

🎯 *Objectives*

- Control blood sugar levels.
- Manage blood pressure.
- Strengthen immunity.
- Provide high biological value nutrients.
- Reduce Physical and Psychological Hunger.
- Promote the process of toxin elimination through the body's natural pathways.
- Stimulate the regeneration process and reversal of damage to cells, tissues, and organs.

RECOMMENDED TIME

4:00 pm - 4:30 pm

Recommendation

At this time, it is important to consume foods that sustain us as this is generally when Physical or Psychological Hunger is most intense.

Proposal

Prepare and drink a juice made of Cucumber, Bitter Melon, Cherry, Chayote, and Lemon.

You can drink two large glasses of this juice until you feel satisfied, as it is a powerful anti-inflammatory and blood sugar regulator.

Important Notes

1. If you are allergic to any ingredient, do not include it; prepare the juice with the other indicated ingredients.

2. The amount of each ingredient should be "to your taste", without forcing the doses.

3. Do not add any sweeteners - sugar or similar - to sweeten the juice.

4. I suggest drinking the juice with a straw, taking a sip every 30 seconds, to make it more palatable.

5. If you have a daily fluid intake restriction due to a condition such as Heart Failure or Renal Insufficiency, only prepare the amount of juice as recommended by your doctor.

#iamfreeofcomplications

dinner

⌖ Objectives

- Avoid spikes in blood sugar levels.
- Strengthen immunity.
- Provide high biological value nutrients.
- Control Physical and Psychological Hunger.
- Stimulate the process of regeneration and reversal of damage to cells, tissues, and organs.

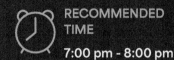

RECOMMENDED TIME

7:00 pm - 8:00 pm

♡ *Recommendation*

Dinner should fulfill two fundamental precepts to stimulate the Body Detoxification process:

1. Be rich in micro and macronutrients.
2. Be easily absorbed by the digestive system.

I propose 5 excellent options

- Barley Stew
- Lentil Soup
- Corn Soup
- Miso Soup
- Millet and Sweet Vegetable Soup

⫰ *Sugestões*

- You should accompany the soup recipes with plenty of raw or steamed vegetable salad.

- It's important to sprinkle Flaxseed, Chia, and Sesame Seeds (powder is better) on top of your meals, after serving them on the table.

✎ *Important Notes*

1. If you are allergic to any ingredient, simply do not use it; prepare the recipes with the other indicated ingredients.

2. You may blend the soup to improve its consistency and taste.

3. You can eat until you feel satisfied, with no restriction on quantity.

4. Avoid drinking water, or any other liquid, during and up to 1 hour after meals.

5. Chew each bite of food between 20 and 50 times until it is completely crushed in your mouth.

#iamfreeofcomplications

tea
normoglycemic

FOOT BATH
RELAXATION AUDIO

Rosemary, Cinnamon, Cow's Foot, and Guava Leaves Tea

🎯 *Objectives*

- Prevent nocturnal hyperglycemia spikes.
- Promote deep, restorative sleep.
- Reduce Physical and Psychological Hunger.
- Strengthen immunity.
- Support the body's natural toxin elimination process.
- Stimulate the regeneration and reversal of damage to cells, tissues, and organs.

RECOMMENDED TIME
9:00 pm - 9:30 pm

Recommendation

Approximately 2 hours after dinner, it is common for blood glucose to start rising as nutrient absorption occurs, including glucose.

Therefore, at this time - 9:00 pm - we should take care to ingest the Normoglycemic Tea to ensure glucose enters the cells, avoiding nocturnal hyperglycemia spikes and acute complications.

Proposal

Prepare the Normoglycemic Tea using Rosemary, Cinnamon, Cow's Foot, and Guava Leaves, adding the juice of one Lemon when the tea is warm.

Prepare the Foot Bath and, while performing it, enjoy your delicious Normoglycemic Tea and listen to a Relaxing Audio accompanied by Breathing Exercises.

Important Notes

1. If you are allergic to any ingredient, simply do not use it; prepare the Tea with the other indicated ingredients.

2. This Normoglycemic Tea is the same one prepared in the morning - to be taken on an empty stomach and as common water before and after meals - so it should be stored in a thermos and consumed, at least, 1 liter throughout the day.

3. If you have a daily liquid intake restriction due to a condition such as Heart Failure or Renal Insufficiency, only prepare the amount of Tea as recommended by your doctor.

4. Do not add any sweetener - sugar or similar - to sweeten the Tea.

5. Never add Lemon juice to hot beverages, as it loses its beneficial properties.

#iamfreeofcomplications

detox
S H O T

Extra Virgin Olive Oil with Lemon

 Objectives

- Detoxify the liver and bile ducts.
- Stimulate intestinal transit.
- Strengthen immunity.
- Support the body's natural toxin elimination process.
- Stimulate the regeneration and reversal of damage to cells, tissues, and organs.

RECOMMENDED TIME

10:00 pm - 10:30 pm

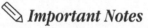 Proposal

After having the Normoglycemic Tea and performing the Foot Bath, it is advisable to prepare a Shot of unrefined Extra Virgin Olive Oil with the juice of one (1) Lemon.

✎ Important Notes

1. If you are allergic to any ingredient, simply do not consume it.

2. This Shot may be unpleasant to taste, so I suggest you take it in one gulp, without "thinking twice," or add a pinch of honey, provided it's been verified that honey consumption does not increase your blood sugar levels.

#iamfreeofcomplications

151

MONDAY
Proposal

Upon waking
Before getting out of bed

1. Listen to the Mental Reprogramming audio.

2. Perform Posture Correction and Hypopressive exercises.

7:00am - 7:30am
Fasting

Start your day by:

1. Drinking the Normoglycemic Tea accompanied by Garlic and Aloe Vera.

2. Doing the Foot Bath with Breathing Exercises.

8:00am - 8:30am
Breakfast

- Natural Cherry Juice with Ginger and Turmeric.

10:00am - 10:30am
Mid-morning snack

- Cucumber Juice with Bitter Melon, Cherry, Chayote, and Lemon.

12:00pm - 1:00pm
Immune-Boosting Shot:
10 minutes before.
Lunch

- Brown Rice with Chickpeas.

- Raw or steamed Vegetable Salad.

4:00pm - 4:30pm
Afternoon Snack

- Cucumber Juice with Bitter Melon, Cherry, Chayote, and Lemon.

7:00pm - 8:00pm
Immune-Boosting Shot:
10 minutes before.
Dinner

- Barley Stew.

- Raw or steamed Vegetable Salad.

9:00pm - 9:30pm
Normoglycemic Tea
Foot Bath
Breathing Exercise

1. Prepare and enjoy your Normoglycemic Tea.

2. Prepare the Foot Bath and, while doing it, enjoy your delicious Normoglycemic Tea and listen to Relaxing Music accompanied by Breathing Exercises.

10:00pm - 10:30pm
Detox Shot

- Take the Detox Shot of unrefined, extra virgin Olive Oil with Lemon juice.

TUESDAY
Proposal

Upon waking
Before getting out of bed

1. Listen to the Mental Reprogramming audio.
2. Perform Posture Correction and Hypopressive exercises.

7:00am - 7:30am
Fasting

Start your day by:

1. Drinking the Normoglycemic Tea accompanied by Garlic and Aloe Vera.
2. Doing the Foot Bath with Breathing Exercises.

8:00am - 8:30am
Breakfast

- Natural Orange Juice with Ginger and Turmeric.

10:00am - 10:30am
Mid-morning snack

- Cucumber Juice with Bitter Melon, Cherry, Chayote, and Lemon.

12:00pm - 1:00pm
*Immune-Boosting Shot:
10 minutes before.
Lunch*

- Brown Rice with Quinoa.
- Raw or steamed Vegetable Salad.

4:00pm - 4:30pm
Afternoon Snack

- Cucumber Juice with Bitter Melon, Cherry, Chayote, and Lemon.

7:00pm - 8:00pm
*Immune-Boosting Shot:
10 minutes before.
Dinner*

- Lentil Soup.
- Raw or steamed Vegetable Salad.

9:00pm - 9:30pm
*Normoglycemic Tea
Foot Bath
Breathing Exercise*

1. Normoglycemic Tea.
2. Prepare the Foot Bath and, while doing it, enjoy your delicious Normoglycemic Tea and listen to Relaxing Music accompanied by Breathing Exercises.

10:00pm - 10:30pm
Detox Shot

- Take the Detox Shot of unrefined, extra virgin Olive Oil with Lemon juice.

#iamfreeofcomplications

153

WEDNESDAY
Proposal

Upon waking
Before getting out of bed

1. Listen to the Mental Reprogramming audio.
2. Perform Posture Correction and Hypopressive exercises.

7:00am - 7:30am
Fasting

Start your day by:

1. Drinking the Normoglycemic Tea accompanied by Garlic and Aloe Vera.
2. Doing the Foot Bath with Breathing Exercises.

8:00am - 8:30am
Breakfast

- Natural Pineapple Juice with Ginger and Turmeric.

10:00am - 10:30am
Mid-morning snack

- Cucumber Juice with Bitter Melon, Cherry, Chayote, and Lemon.

12:00pm – 1:00pm
Immune-Boosting Shot:
10 minutes before.
Lunch

- Whole Grain Rice with Corn.
- Raw or steamed Vegetable Salad.

4:00pm - 4:30pm
Afternoon Snack

- Cucumber Juice with Bitter Melon, Cherry, Chayote, and Lemon.

7:00pm - 8:00pm
Immune-Boosting Shot:
10 minutes before.
Dinner

- Corn Soup.
- Raw or steamed Vegetable Salad.

9:00pm - 9:30pm
Normoglycemic Tea
Foot Bath
Breathing Exercise

1. Normoglycemic Tea.
2. Prepare the Foot Bath and, while doing it, enjoy your delicious Normoglycemic Tea and listen to Relaxing Music accompanied by Breathing Exercises.

10:00pm - 10:30pm
Detox Shot

- Take the Detox Shot of unrefined, extra virgin Olive Oil with Lemon juice.

THURSDAY
Proposal

Upon waking
Before getting out of bed

1. Listen to the Mental Reprogramming audio.
2. Perform Posture Correction and Hypopressive exercises.

7:00am - 7:30am
Fasting

Start your day by:

1. Drinking the Normoglycemic Tea accompanied by Garlic and Aloe Vera.
2. Doing the Foot Bath with Breathing Exercises.

8:00am - 8:30am
Breakfast

- Natural Cherry Juice with Ginger and Turmeric.

10:00am - 10:30am
Mid-morning snack

- Cucumber Juice with Bitter Melon, Cherry, Chayote, and Lemon.

12:00pm – 1:00pm
Immune-Boosting Shot:
10 minutes before.
Lunch

- Integral Rice with Lentils.
- Raw or steamed Vegetable Salad.

4:00pm - 4:30pm
Afternoon Snack

- Cucumber Juice with Bitter Melon, Cherry, Chayote, and Lemon.

7:00pm - 8:00pm
Immune-Boosting Shot:
10 minutes before.
Dinner

- Miso Soup.
- Raw or steamed Vegetable Salad.

9:00pm - 9:30pm
Normoglycemic Tea
Foot Bath
Breathing Exercise

1. Normoglycemic Tea.
2. Prepare the Foot Bath and, while doing it, enjoy your delicious Normoglycemic Tea and listen to Relaxing Music accompanied by Breathing Exercises.

10:00pm - 10:30pm
Detox Shot

- Take the Detox Shot of unrefined, extra virgin Olive Oil with Lemon juice.

#iamfreeofcomplications

155

FRIDAY
Proposal

Upon waking
Before getting out of bed

1. Listen to the Mental Reprogramming audio.

2. Perform Posture Correction and Hypopressive exercises.

7:00am - 7:30am
Fasting

Start your day by:

1. Drinking the Normoglycemic Tea accompanied by Garlic and Aloe Vera.

2. Doing the Foot Bath with Breathing Exercises.

8:00am - 8:30am
Breakfast

- Natural Orange Juice with Ginger and Turmeric.

10:00am - 10:30am
Mid-morning snack

- Cucumber Juice with Bitter Melon, Cherry, Chayote, and Lemon.

12:00pm - 1:00pm
Immune-Boosting Shot:
10 minutes before.
Lunch

- Brown Rice with Millet or Barley.

- Raw or steamed Vegetable Salad.

4:00pm - 4:30pm
Afternoon Snack

- Cucumber Juice with Bitter Melon, Cherry, Chayote, and Lemon.

7:00pm - 8:00pm
Immune-Boosting Shot:
10 minutes before.
Dinner

- Millet Soup and Sweet Vegetables.

- Raw or steamed Vegetable Salad.

9:00pm - 9:30pm
Normoglycemic Tea
Foot Bath
Breathing Exercise

1. Normoglycemic Tea.

2. Prepare the Foot Bath and, while doing it, enjoy your delicious Normoglycemic Tea and listen to Relaxing Music accompanied by Breathing Exercises.

10:00pm - 10:30pm
Detox Shot

- Take the Detox Shot of unrefined, extra virgin Olive Oil with Lemon juice.

SATURDAY AND SUNDAY
Proposal

Upon waking
Before getting out of bed

1. Listen to the Mental Reprogramming audio.
2. Perform Posture Correction and Hypopressive exercises.

7:00am - 7:30am
Fasting

Start your day by:

1. Drinking the Normoglycemic Tea accompanied by Garlic and Aloe Vera.
2. Doing the Foot Bath with Breathing Exercises.

8:00am - 8:30am
Breakfast

- You can choose from the three options of Natural Juice with Ginger and Turmeric.

10:00am - 10:30am
Mid-morning snack

- Cucumber Juice with Bitter Melon, Cherry, Chayote, and Lemon.

12:00pm - 1:00pm
Immune-Boosting Shot:
10 minutes before.
Lunch

- You can choose from the 5 options of Brown Rice.
- Raw or steamed Vegetable Salad.

4:00pm - 4:30pm
Afternoon Snack

- Cucumber Juice with Bitter Melon, Cherry, Chayote, and Lemon.

7:00pm - 8:00pm
Immune-Boosting Shot:
10 minutes before.
Dinner

- You can choose from the 5 options of Soups.
- Raw or steamed Vegetable Salad.

9:00pm - 9:30pm
Normoglycemic Tea
Foot Bath
Breathing Exercise

1. Normoglycemic Tea.
2. Prepare the Foot Bath and, while doing it, enjoy your delicious Normoglycemic Tea and listen to Relaxing Music accompanied by Breathing Exercises.

10:00pm - 10:30pm
Detox Shot

- Take the Detox Shot of unrefined, extra virgin Olive Oil with Lemon juice.

#iamfreeofcomplications

157

What to Do After the

30 DAYS

Detox?

As part of a nutritional reeducation program, one of the goals of this method is for you to adopt a Healthy Lifestyle, so our main suggestion is to embrace this system for life with some adjustments to have more variety in your diet.

I'll list the modifications you can make after the 30 days of Body Detox in order of importance.

Suggestions After the 30 Days

Regarding the Normoglycemic Tea

1. From Monday to Friday, prepare the Normoglycemic Tea with all the ingredients and drink 1 liter per day at the recommended times.

2. On Saturday and Sunday, prepare the same amount of Normoglycemic Tea but with only one of the ingredients and lemon.

Regarding the Foot Bath

You can do it on alternate days and only for 10 minutes at the recommended times (morning and night).

Regarding Breakfast

I suggest you keep the same juice recommendations, and if you want to add some solid food, an Omelette (with two eggs, onion, and chives to taste),

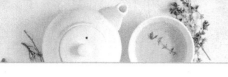
prepared in a non-stick pan or using extra virgin Olive Oil, is an excellent option.

Regarding Morning and Afternoon Snacks

The Cucumber Juice is something you should take for life as you once did with milk, which did not provide any nutrients.

If you wish, you can also drink the Juices Indicated for Breakfast during the Snacks.

Regarding Lunch

I suggest you keep the same recipes and add white meats such as chicken, fish, and rabbit three (3) times a week and eggs four (4) times a week.

Regarding Dinner

I suggest you maintain the same recipes and add white meats such as chicken, fish, and rabbit five (5) times a week and red meats once (1) a week.

Regarding the Detox Shot

You can repeat a cycle of taking it for 5 days and then take 25 days off.

Regarding the Mental Reprogramming Audio and the Hypopressive and Breathing Exercises

I suggest incorporating them into your daily routine as they are excellent health allies.

Dr. Quesada's Advice

1. Following the naturalist proposals in this book will always bring you peace of mind, confidence, and health.

2. When in doubt, it's always recommended to consult your doctor. All the suggestions made in this book do not fully or partially substitute for your doctor's advice.

#iamfreeofcomplications

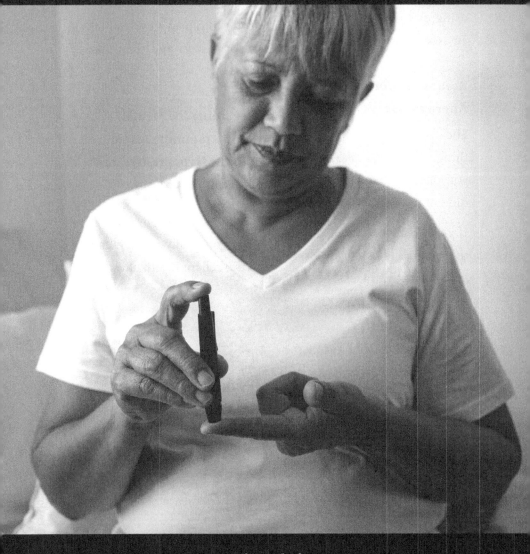

the end of
**DIABETES
MELLITUS**

CHAPTER 8

CONTROL
SYSTEM

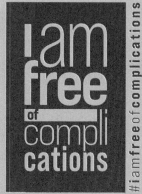

i am
free
of
compli
cations

#iamfreeofcomplications

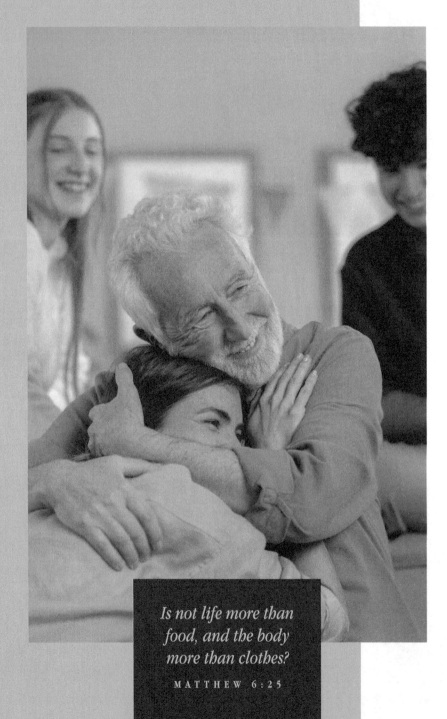

the *end of*
DIABETES MELLITUS

Is not life more than food, and the body more than clothes?

MATTHEW 6:25

Therapist, in the following pages, you will find 3 types of control that you must keep, daily and exhaustively, for the time you are following the recommendations of this book:

- Blood glucose control at 4 times of the day.
- Control of daily recommendations.
- Control of symptom evolution.

PRACTICAL TIPS FOR EFFECTIVE CONTROL

1. **Set alarms:** set alerts on your phone or watch to remind you when to check your blood glucose. This will help you maintain a regular schedule and not forget the measurements.

2. **Be disciplined:** when your phone alarm goes off, make an effort to do the check at that moment.

3. **Carry testing supplies with you:** always carry your glucose meter, test strips, and a lancet, especially if you're out of the house or at work. This will allow you to test even when you're not at home.

4. **Share your results:** share your blood glucose records, symptom evolution, etc., with your family and friends, including your primary care physician.

5. **Day completed:** never go to bed without having recorded your results in the Control Tables.

Following these practical tips and keeping an organized record, you will have absolute control of your progress. Remember the old and wise saying: *"I am the captain of my destiny..."*

#iamfreeofcomplications

BLOOD GLUCOSE CONTROL

Multiple scientific studies concluded that daily blood glucose measurements at specific times of the day contribute to the proper control of diabetes mellitus and reduce the complications and mortality of this disease.

Performed 4 times a day, it is essential for effective DM management and to improve life prognosis.

These controls provide real-time information to make decisions about diet, medication, and lifestyle, contributing to improving the quality of life for people with diabetes, while reducing the risk of acute and chronic complications.

The 4 blood glucose controls
- Fasting Blood Glucose

Postprandial Blood Glucose
- 2 hours after Breakfast
- 2 hours after Lunch
- 2 hours after Dinner

FASTING BLOOD GLUCOSE

It is a marker of the effect of the foods we eat at dinner or after it.

- **Fasting Blood Glucose:** 80-130 mg/dl (4.4-7.2 mmol/L)

If blood glucose is elevated in the morning, above 130 mg/dl, it means we need to modify what we are having for dinner and/or be cautious with food intake after Dinner.

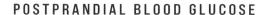

POSTPRANDIAL BLOOD GLUCOSE

Known as postprandial glucose, it shows the body's response to the foods we ingest (main meals of the day).

- **Postprandial glucose:** <180 mg/dl (10 mmol/L)

If, 2 hours after eating, the blood glucose remains above 180 mg/dl, it means that the foods we are consuming do not favor the process of control and reversal of diabetes damage.

Test	Control Range
Fasting Blood Glucose	80-130 mg/dl (4.4-7.2 mmol/L)
Postprandial Blood Glucose *	<180 mg/dl (10 mmol/L)

* Up to 2 hours after the main meals of the day.

 Important Notes

1. The most important blood glucose readings of the day are those you measure Fasting and 2 hours after Dinner. These measurements are essential in your daily control because most of the acute complications of diabetes occur at night, while you are sleeping.

2. You should never go to sleep with blood glucose above 180 mg/dl because, as mentioned before, most of the acute complications of diabetes develop while you are sleeping.

3. In case your blood glucose is above 180 mg/dl in the control 2 hours after Dinner, it's important to prepare the Tea indicated for 9:00 pm and drink it, you can even have more than one glass.

4. When, in the blood glucose controls, you detect elevated levels (greater than 180 mg/dl), I suggest identifying if you present any accompanying symptoms and note it on your symptom evolution sheet.

In the following tables, record the date and note the blood glucose results (mg/dl or mmol/l).

#iamfreeofcomplications

TABLE 1 | DAILY GLYCEMIA CONTROL

SUNDAY
DATE   /   /

Fasting	
2 hours after Breakfast	
2 hours after Lunch	
2 hours after Dinner	

MONDAY
DATE   /   /

Fasting	
2 hours after Breakfast	
2 hours after Lunch	
2 hours after Dinner	

TUESDAY
DATE   /   /

Fasting	
2 hours after Breakfast	
2 hours after Lunch	
2 hours after Dinner	

WEDNESDAY
DATE   /   /

Fasting	
2 hours after Breakfast	
2 hours after Lunch	
2 hours after Dinner	

THURSDAY
DATE   /   /

Fasting	
2 hours after Breakfast	
2 hours after Lunch	
2 hours after Dinner	

FRIDAY
DATE   /   /

Fasting	
2 hours after Breakfast	
2 hours after Lunch	
2 hours after Dinner	

SATURDAY
DATE   /   /

Fasting	
2 hours after Breakfast	
2 hours after Lunch	
2 hours after Dinner	

NORMAL VALUES

Fasting Glucose: 80-130 mg/dl (4.4-7.2 mmol/L)	Postprandial Glucose: <180 mg/dl (10 mmol/L)

SUNDAY
DATA

- Fasting
- 2 hours after Breakfast
- 2 hours after Lunch
- 2 hours after Dinner

MONDAY
DATA

- Fasting
- 2 hours after Breakfast
- 2 hours after Lunch
- 2 hours after Dinner

TUESDAY
DATA

- Fasting
- 2 hours after Breakfast
- 2 hours after Lunch
- 2 hours after Dinner

WEDNESDAY
DATA

- Fasting
- 2 hours after Breakfast
- 2 hours after Lunch
- 2 hours after Dinner

THURSDAY
DATA

- Fasting
- 2 hours after Breakfast
- 2 hours after Lunch
- 2 hours after Dinner

FRIDAY
DATA

- Fasting
- 2 hours after Breakfast
- 2 hours after Lunch
- 2 hours after Dinner

SATURDAY
DATA

- Fasting
- 2 hours after Breakfast
- 2 hours after Lunch
- 2 hours after Dinner

#iamfreeofcomplications

NORMAL VALUES

Fasting Glucose: 80-130 mg/dl (4.4-7.2 mmol/L) | Postprandial Glucose: <180 mg/dl (10 mmol/L)

TABLE 1 | DAILY GLYCEMIA CONTROL

SUNDAY
DATE   /   /

- Fasting
- 2 hours after Breakfast
- 2 hours after Lunch
- 2 hours after Dinner

MONDAY
DATE   /   /

- Fasting
- 2 hours after Breakfast
- 2 hours after Lunch
- 2 hours after Dinner

TUESDAY
DATE   /   /

- Fasting
- 2 hours after Breakfast
- 2 hours after Lunch
- 2 hours after Dinner

WEDNESDAY
DATE   /   /

- Fasting
- 2 hours after Breakfast
- 2 hours after Lunch
- 2 hours after Dinner

THURSDAY
DATE   /   /

- Fasting
- 2 hours after Breakfast
- 2 hours after Lunch
- 2 hours after Dinner

FRIDAY
DATE   /   /

- Fasting
- 2 hours after Breakfast
- 2 hours after Lunch
- 2 hours after Dinner

SATURDAY
DATE   /   /

- Fasting
- 2 hours after Breakfast
- 2 hours after Lunch
- 2 hours after Dinner

NORMAL VALUES

Fasting Glucose: 80-130 mg/dl (4.4-7.2 mmol/L)	Postprandial Glucose: <180 mg/dl (10 mmol/L)

SUNDAY

DATA

- Fasting
- 2 hours after Breakfast
- 2 hours after Lunch
- 2 hours after Dinner

MONDAY

DATA

- Fasting
- 2 hours after Breakfast
- 2 hours after Lunch
- 2 hours after Dinner

TUESDAY

DATA

- Fasting
- 2 hours after Breakfast
- 2 hours after Lunch
- 2 hours after Dinner

WEDNESDAY

DATA

- Fasting
- 2 hours after Breakfast
- 2 hours after Lunch
- 2 hours after Dinner

THURSDAY

DATA

- Fasting
- 2 hours after Breakfast
- 2 hours after Lunch
- 2 hours after Dinner

FRIDAY

DATA

- Fasting
- 2 hours after Breakfast
- 2 hours after Lunch
- 2 hours after Dinner

SATURDAY

DATA

- Fasting
- 2 hours after Breakfast
- 2 hours after Lunch
- 2 hours after Dinner

#iamfreeofcomplications

NORMAL VALUES

Fasting Glucose: 80-130 mg/dl (4.4-7.2 mmol/L)	Postprandial Glucose: <180 mg/dl (10 mmol/L)

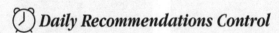

Daily Recommendations Control

It's extremely important as it demonstrates your level of discipline and commitment to your health and your desire to be free from the symptoms, medications, risks, and complications of this disease.

In the following tables, record the Date and mark the Recommendations completed daily.

TABLE 2 | CONTROL OF DAILY RECOMMENDATIONS

	sum	mon	tue	wed	thu	fri	sun
Upon waking *Before Getting Up* *Audio-Exercises*	✓	☐	☐	☐	☐	☐	☐
7:00 am - 7:30 am *Fasting*	☐	☐	☐	☐	☐	☐	☐
8:00 am - 8:30 am *Breakfast*	☐	☐	☐	☐	☐	☐	☐
10:00 am - 10:30 am *Snack*	☐	☐	☐	☐	☐	☐	☐
12:00 pm - 1:00 pm *Immunostimulant Shot* *Lunch*	☐ ☐	☐ ☐	☐ ☐	☐ ☐	☐ ☐	☐ ☐	☐ ☐
4:00 pm - 4:30 pm *Snack*	☐	☐	☐	☐	☐	☐	☐
7:00 pm - 8:00 pm *Immunostimulant Shot* *Dinner*	☐ ☐	☐ ☐	☐ ☐	☐ ☐	☐ ☐	☐ ☐	☐ ☐
9:00 pm - 9:30 pm *Normoglycemic Tea* *Pediluvium*	☐	☐	☐	☐	☐	☐	☐
10:00 pm - 10:30 pm *Detox Shot*	☐	☐	☐	☐	☐	☐	☐

#iamfreeofcomplications

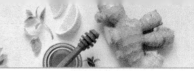

TABLE 2 | CONTROL OF DAILY RECOMMENDATIONS

	sum	mon	tue	wed	thu	fri	sun
Upon waking *Before Getting Up* *Audio-Exercises*	☐	☐	☐	☐	☐	☐	☐
7:00 am - 7:30 am *Fasting*	☐	☐	☐	☐	☐	☐	☐
8:00 am - 8:30 am *Breakfast*	☐	☐	☐	☐	☐	☐	☐
10:00 am - 10:30 am *Snack*	☐	☐	☐	☐	☐	☐	☐
12:00 pm - 1:00 pm *Immunostimulant Shot* *Lunch*	☐☐	☐☐	☐☐	☐☐	☐☐	☐☐	☐☐
4:00 pm - 4:30 pm *Snack*	☐	☐	☐	☐	☐	☐	☐
7:00 pm - 8:00 pm *Immunostimulant Shot* *Dinner*	☐☐	☐☐	☐☐	☐☐	☐☐	☐☐	☐☐
9:00 pm - 9:30 pm *Normoglycemic Tea* *Pediluvium*	☐	☐	☐	☐	☐	☐	☐
10:00 pm - 10:30 pm *Detox Shot*	☐	☐	☐	☐	☐	☐	☐

TABLE 2 | CONTROL OF DAILY RECOMMENDATIONS

	sum	mon	tue	wed	thu	fri	sun
Upon waking *Before Getting Up Audio-Exercises*	☐	☐	☐	☐	☐	☐	☐
7:00 am - 7:30 am *Fasting*	☐	☐	☐	☐	☐	☐	☐
8:00 am - 8:30 am *Breakfast*	☐	☐	☐	☐	☐	☐	☐
10:00 am - 10:30 am *Snack*	☐	☐	☐	☐	☐	☐	☐
12:00 pm - 1:00 pm *Immunostimulant Shot* *Lunch*	☐☐	☐☐	☐☐	☐☐	☐☐	☐☐	☐☐
4:00 pm - 4:30 pm *Snack*	☐	☐	☐	☐	☐	☐	☐
7:00 pm - 8:00 pm *Immunostimulant Shot* *Dinner*	☐☐	☐☐	☐☐	☐☐	☐☐	☐☐	☐☐
9:00 pm - 9:30 pm *Normoglycemic Tea* *Pediluvium*	☐	☐	☐	☐	☐	☐	☐
10:00 pm - 10:30 pm *Detox Shot*	☐	☐	☐	☐	☐	☐	☐

#iamfreeofcomplications

TABLE 2 | CONTROL OF DAILY RECOMMENDATIONS

	sum	mon	tue	wed	thu	fri	sun
Upon waking *Before Getting Up* *Audio-Exercises*	☐	☐	☐	☐	☐	☐	☐
7:00 am - 7:30 am *Fasting*	☐	☐	☐	☐	☐	☐	☐
8:00 am - 8:30 am *Breakfast*	☐	☐	☐	☐	☐	☐	☐
10:00 am - 10:30 am *Snack*	☐	☐	☐	☐	☐	☐	☐
12:00 pm - 1:00 pm *Immunostimulant Shot* *Lunch*	☐☐	☐☐	☐☐	☐☐	☐☐	☐☐	☐☐
4:00 pm - 4:30 pm *Snack*	☐	☐	☐	☐	☐	☐	☐
7:00 pm - 8:00 pm *Immunostimulant Shot* *Dinner*	☐☐	☐☐	☐☐	☐☐	☐☐	☐☐	☐☐
9:00 pm - 9:30 pm *Normoglycemic Tea* *Pediluvium*	☐	☐	☐	☐	☐	☐	☐
10:00 pm - 10:30 pm *Detox Shot*	☐	☐	☐	☐	☐	☐	☐

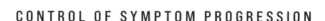

CONTROL OF SYMPTOM PROGRESSION

By making a correct diagnosis and monitoring the progression of symptoms, you will be able to know how you are evolving, whether the treatment is effective, and whether your body is responding favorably.

The most common symptoms of diabetes mellitus were described in the General Concepts chapter.

Classification of symptoms according to their intensity:

Mild: if it does not interfere with the ability to perform daily activities.

Moderate: when it hinders these activities.

Severe: when it interferes, even, with rest.

In the following tables, record the symptoms present, the date, their intensity, and their evolution according to the classification of:

- Mild
- Moderate
- Severe

Always start by recording the symptom that most limits your quality of life.

#iamfreeofcomplications

TABLE 3 | CONTROL OF SYMPTOM PROGRESSION

SYMPTOMS	DATE / / Intensity	DATE / / Intensity	DATE / / Intensity

Place the symbol in each Control according to the Symptom Evolution

↑ Increased
+– Remained the same
↓ Decreased
⊗ Disappeared

DATE / /	DATE / /	DATE / /	DATE / /
Intensity	*Intensity*	*Intensity*	*Intensity*

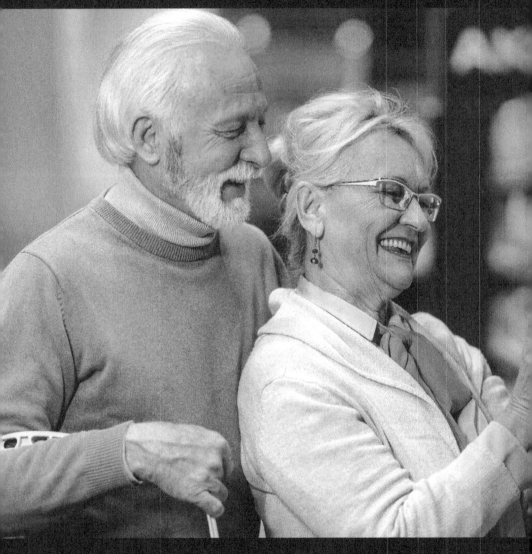

the *end* of
**DIABETES
MELLITUS**

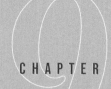

LIST
SHOPPING

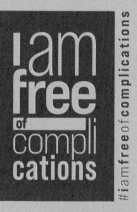

i am
free
of
compli
cations

#iamfreeofcomplications

@draldenquesada.es

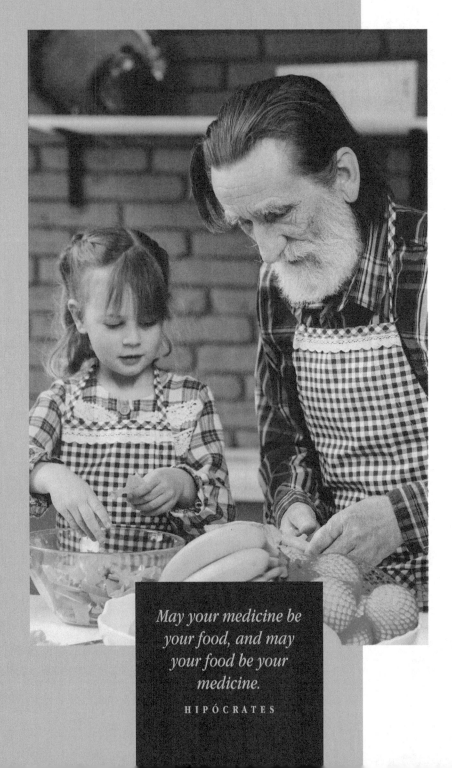

the end of
DIABETES
MELLITUS

*May your medicine be
your food, and may
your food be your
medicine.*

HIPÓCRATES

D ear Therapist, I am sharing with you a powerful Shopping List for when you go to the market.

It's important that you only buy what is indicated on this List as this is where your process of bodily detoxification and dietary re-education begins to create new healthy behavior patterns.

It is not necessary to buy all the products; however, all the indicated products, if properly grown and harvested, are rich in micro and macronutrients.

Keep in mind that some products are repeated in the recipes, and that cucumber and tomato are fruits, so they are not recommended for preparing the Vegetable Salad.

Happy shopping!

#iamfreeofcomplications

NORMOGLYCEMIC
tea

Ingredients

- ☐ Rosemary (leaves)
- ☐ Cinnamon (stick or powder)
- ☐ Guava (leaves)
- ☐ Bauhinia spp. (pata de vaca)- (leaves)
- ☐ Turmeric (grated or in powder)
- ☐ Ginger (grated or in powder)
- ☐ Lemon

Others

- ☐ Garlic
- ☐ Aloe vera

IMMUNE-BOOSTING
shot

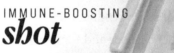

Ingredients

- ☐ Apple cider vinegar
- ☐ Propolis

DETOX
shot

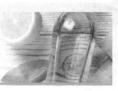

Ingredients

- ☐ Extra Virgin Olive Oil (unrefined)
- ☐ Lemon

RECIPES
sucos

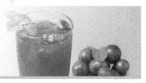

Ingredients

- ☐ Cherry
- ☐ Apple
- ☐ Orange
- ☐ Pineapple
- ☐ Ginger (grated or in powder)
- ☐ Turmeric (grated or in powder)

CUCUMBER
vitamin

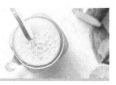

Ingredients

- ☐ Cucumber (any variety)
- ☐ Cundeamor (Momordica charantia)
- ☐ Chayote
- ☐ Cherry
- ☐ Lemon

#iamfreeofcomplications

LUNCH

brown rice
RECIPES

vegetable
RECIPES

Ingredients

- [ ] Organic Brown Rice
- [ ] Chickpeas
- [ ] Lentils
- [ ] Corn
- [ ] Millet or Barley
- [ ] Quinoa
- [ ] Onion
- [ ] Garlic
- [ ] Ora pro nobis
- [ ] Cauliflower
- [ ] Broccoli
- [ ] Green pepper (or red)
- [ ] Sea salt (or unrefined coarse salt)

Ingredients

- [ ] Cabbage
- [ ] Broccoli
- [ ] Cauliflower
- [ ] Spinach
- [ ] Watercress
- [ ] Leek
- [ ] Carrot
- [ ] Daikon
- [ ] Turnip
- [ ] Parsley
- [ ] Chives
- [ ] Dandelion leaves
- [ ] Lemon

soup
RECIPES

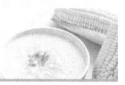

Ingredients

- [ ] Barley
- [ ] Green or brown lentils
- [ ] Fresh corn on the cob or kernels
- [ ] Barley miso
- [ ] Millet
- [ ] Garlic
- [ ] Onion
- [ ] Cauliflower
- [ ] Broccoli
- [ ] Cabbage
- [ ] Carrot
- [ ] Zucchini
- [ ] Spinach
- [ ] Celery
- [ ] Shoyu
- [ ] Leek
- [ ] Chives
- [ ] Parsley
- [ ] Shiitake Mushroom
- [ ] Wakame
- [ ] Green or red pepper
- [ ] Ora pro nobis (Pereskia aculeata)
- [ ] Sea salt (or unrefined coarse salt)

foot
BATH

Ingredients

- [ ] Sea salt (or unrefined coarse salt)
- [ ] Ginger (grated or in powder)
- [ ] Basin

DINNER

#iamfreeofcomplications

185

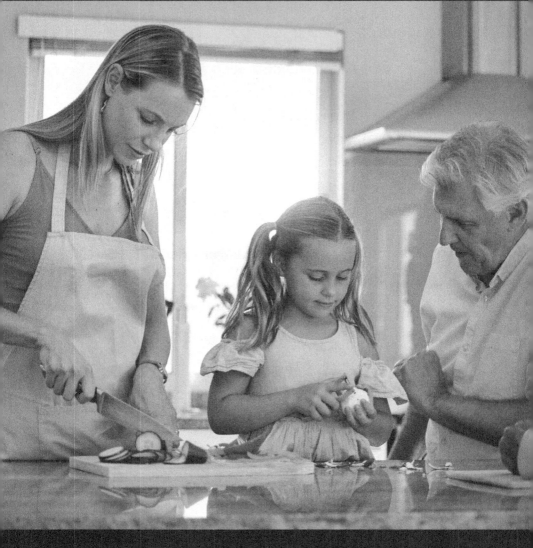

the *end* of
DIABETES
MELLITUS

CHAPTER 10

RECIPES AND
PROCE
DURES

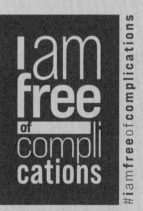

i am
free
of
compli
cations

#iamfreeofcomplications

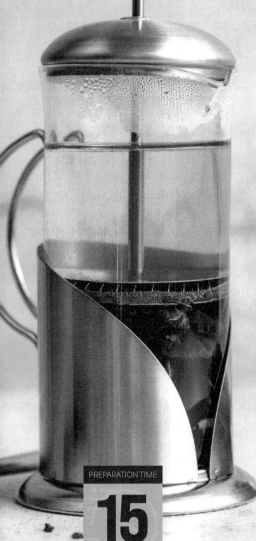

normoglycemic TEA

📖 INGREDIENTS

- [ ] **Water:** 1½ liters (1500 ml)
- [ ] **Turmeric:** grated or powder
- [ ] **Ginger:** grated or powder
- [ ] **Rosemary:** 2 tablespoons of dried leaves
- [ ] **Cinnamon:** 1 stick or 1 tablespoon in powder
- [ ] **Guava:** 10 g of dried leaves
- [ ] **Bauhinia forficata (Pata de Vaca):** 2 tablespoons of dried leaves
- [ ] **Lemon:** juice of one (1) unit

☕ PREPARATION METHOD

1. Place the water on the heat with the Cinnamon stick, Ginger, and Turmeric.

2. Bring the water to a boil for 1 minute, then add the Rosemary, Guava, and Pata de Vaca leaves. Turn off the heat and, with the pot covered, let it steep for 5 to 10 minutes.

3. Strain the Tea and then add the juice of 1 Lemon when the Tea is lukewarm -never hot-.

PREPARATION TIME

15
minutes

RECOMMENDEDS TIMES

- **7:00 am.** Have a cup on an empty stomach

- **11:30 pm.** Have a cup 30 minutes before Lunch

- **2:00 pm.** Have a cup 2 hours after Lunch

- **7:30 pm.** Have a cup 30 minutes before Dinner

- **9:00 pm.** Have a cup 2 hours after Dinner

    You should drink 1 ½ liters per day of this Normoglycemic Tea, so I suggest you carry it to your work in a thermos and drink it like regular water, always 30 minutes before and 2 hours after the main meals of the day.

IMPORTANT NOTES

1. If you have a known allergy to Rosemary, Cinnamon, Pata de Vaca, or any other product indicated for preparing the Tea, simply do not buy or use it, but DO NOT STOP MAKING it with the other ingredients.

2. In addition to being used as Tea, Rosemary can be used as an aromatic herb to season foods.

ROSEMARY IS NOT RECOMMENDED FOR:

- People hypersensitive or allergic to its components.

- Should not be used by children under 12 years of age, pregnant or breastfeeding women.

- Those with an allergy to aspirin, as the spice contains salicylate, a component similar to the medication.

- People with liver diseases or gallbladder issues. In the latter case, this is because the Tea can worsen the disease and increase its symptoms.

- Finally, if you have any seizure disorder, it is also not recommended.

CINNAMON IS NOT RECOMMENDED FOR:

- People allergic to its components.

- Should not be used by children under 12 years of age, pregnant or breastfeeding women.

- People with high blood pressure as it may increase pressure in patients sensitive to the components of Cinnamon.

BAUHINIA FORFICATA IS NOT RECOMMENDED FOR:

- People allergic to its components.

- Should not be used by children under 12 years of age, pregnant or breastfeeding women.

#iamfreeofcomplications

Eating GARLIC
on an Empty Stomach

While garlic is a staple ingredient in our meals, to take advantage of its health properties, it's proven that the best option is to consume it raw and on an empty stomach.

Raw garlic ensures a higher intake of Allicin, the main organosulfur compound to which medicinal properties are attributed.

It has been observed that the concentration of Allicin decreases significantly during cooking and increases when garlic is cut or crushed.

PREPARATION TIME

10 minutes

HOW TO CONSUME GARLIC

In small slices, finely cut, that can easily pass through the throat without causing discomfort.

Important note: Consuming the whole garlic clove, without cutting it, will have little health benefits.

RECOMMENDED TIME

- **7:00 am.** Always on an empty stomach, accompanied by sips of Normoglycemic Tea.

PREPARATION METHOD

1. Select a medium-sized garlic clove.
2. Ensure the garlic is fresh. An overly old garlic clove may not have the necessary amount of beneficial compounds.
3. Peel and slice the garlic into very small cubes.
4. Let it sit for 1 to 3 minutes before consuming.

BENEFITS OF GARLIC

- **Weight Loss:** It has thermogenic properties that can speed up metabolism and weight loss.

- **Antibacterial Properties:** It has antibacterial and antiviral actions, helping to prevent and treat infections.

- **Reduces Blood Pressure:** Some studies suggest that garlic can help reduce blood pressure, especially in people who suffer from this condition.

- **Improves Lipid Profile:** It helps reduce levels of LDL cholesterol (bad cholesterol) and slightly increase HDL (good cholesterol).

- **Antioxidant Properties:** Contains antioxidants that help protect cells against damage caused by free radicals.

- **Prevention of Heart Diseases:** Some studies suggest that frequent consumption of garlic can help reduce clot formation and arteriosclerosis.

- **Strengthens the Immune System:** Regularly consuming garlic strengthens the immune system and helps fight infections.

- **Reduction of the Risk of Certain Types of Cancer:** Regular consumption is also associated with a lower risk of developing certain types of cancer.

- **Prevents Osteoporosis:** Some studies have suggested that garlic could benefit bone health and prevent osteoporosis.

- **Stimulates Cognitive Function:** The antioxidants present in garlic help prevent neurodegenerative diseases.

IMPORTANT NOTES

1. If you have a known allergy to garlic, do not consume it.

2. Consuming large amounts of garlic on an empty stomach could cause stomach irritation. Limit the amount to one medium-sized garlic clove to prevent possible side effects.

3. You should ingest the garlic without chewing it, i.e., swallow it accompanied by sips of Normoglycemic Tea, hence it's important to cut it into very small cubes.

#iamfreeofcomplications

191

ALOE VERA

on an empty stomach

 STEPS TO PREPARE THE "CRYSTALS"

1. Cut a leaf of Aloe Vera at the base with a knife.

2. Cut off the leaf's lateral edges that contain small thorns.

3. Thoroughly wash the leaves with plenty of water.

4. Peel off the leaf's skin and discard it.

5. Remove the yellow layer underneath the skin (it's irritating and very bitter).

6. Wash again with plenty of water, until all the gelatinous liquid is removed, and only the crystals remain, i.e., the gelatinous and transparent substance inside the leaves.

7. Cut the crystals into small squares - the size of a capsule - and place them in the refrigerator (you can use ice cube trays).

Aloe Vera, also known as Sábila, is one of the most well-known medicinal plants globally and can be consumed in various ways.

It's possible to ingest this herb in juices, teas, or even in small pieces -capsules-.

 HOW TO CONSUME ALOE VERA

In small "capsules," that can easily pass through the throat without causing discomfort.

 RECOMMENDED TIME

- **7:00 am.** Always on an empty stomach, accompanied by sips of Normoglycemic Tea.

PREPARATION TIME

10
minutes

BENEFITS OF ALOE VERA

- **Antioxidant Properties:** contains antioxidant substances that help protect the body's cells against oxidative stress and premature aging.

- **Strengthening the Immune System:** some components of Aloe Vera have a stimulating effect on the immune system, helping to strengthen the body's defenses.

- **Natural Anti-inflammatory:** its anti-inflammatory properties help reduce inflammation in various parts of the body.

- **Skin Hydration:** known for its ability to hydrate the skin, helping to keep it soft and flexible.

- **Wound Healing:** Aloe Vera gel accelerates the healing process of wounds, sunburns, and cuts, due to its anti-inflammatory and regenerative properties.

- **Stimulates Digestion:** consuming Aloe Vera juice helps improve digestive problems and promote intestinal regularity.

- **Treatment of Skin Conditions:** beneficial in cases of skin conditions like eczema, psoriasis, and acne, due to its anti-inflammatory and antimicrobial properties.

- **Promotes Hair Growth:** proven effective in improving scalp health and stimulating hair growth.

IMPORTANT NOTES

1. If you have a known allergy to Aloe Vera, do not consume it.

2. If you have any degree or suspicion of Renal Insufficiency, do not consume Aloe Vera.

3. Consume Aloe Vera for 30 days.

4. Consuming large amounts of Aloe Vera on an empty stomach could cause stomach discomfort. Limit the amount to two capsules to prevent possible side effects.

5. You should ingest the Aloe Vera capsules without chewing them, accompanied by sips of Normoglycemic Tea, hence the capsules should not be too large.

#iamfreeofcomplications

BREAKFAST

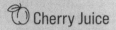 Cherry Juice   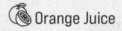 Orange Juice   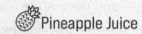 Pineapple Juice

cherry
JUICE

Ingredients

- ☐ **Cherries:** 2 cups
- ☐ **Apple:** 1 unit
- ☐ **Ginger:** to taste (grated or powder)
- ☐ **Turmeric:** to taste (grated or powder)
- ☐ **Water:** 250 ml

IMPORTANT NOTES

1. If you are allergic to any component suggested in the recipe, simply do not add it to the preparation.

2. You can drink two large glasses of any of the juices until you feel satisfied, as they are potent anti-inflammatory agents and provide vitamins and minerals.

3. All ingredients should be "to your taste," without forcing the doses.

PREPARATION METHOD

1. Thoroughly wash the Cherries and Apple with plenty of Water.

2. In a Blender, place the Cherries, Apple, Water, Ginger, and Turmeric, and blend everything until homogeneous.

3. If preferred, strain through a medium-mesh strainer, pressing to extract the liquid and discard the solids.

4. You may add one (1) ice cube to slightly cool the juice.

5. Consume immediately.

RECOMMENDED TIME

- 8:00 am - 8:30 am.

PREPARATION TIME

10 minutes

orange
JUICE

Pineapple
JUICE

Ingredients

- **Oranges:** 2 units
- **Cherries:** 2 cups
- **Ginger:** to taste (grated or powder)
- **Turmeric:** to taste (grated or powder)

Ingredients

- **Pineapple:** quantity to taste
- **Cherries:** 2 cups
- **Ginger:** to taste (grated or powder)
- **Turmeric:** to taste (grated or powder)
- **Water:** 250 ml

 PREPARATION METHOD

1. Thoroughly wash the Oranges and Cherries with plenty of Water.
2. Cut the Oranges in half and squeeze them.
3. Collect the juice in a clean container, including the pulp, and discard the seeds.
4. Blend the Cherries in a blender with the Turmeric and Ginger and, once blended, add to a preferably glass jug along with the Orange juice.
5. You may add one (1) ice cube to slightly cool the juice.
6. Consume immediately.

 PREPARATION METHOD

1. Thoroughly wash the Cherries with plenty of Water.
2. In a Blender, place the Pineapple slices with Water, Cherries, Ginger, and Turmeric, and blend everything until homogeneous.
3. If preferred, strain through a medium-mesh strainer, pressing to extract the liquid and discard the solids.
4. You may add an ice cube to slightly cool the juice.
5. Consume immediately.

#iamfreeofcomplications

CUCUMBER
juice

Ingredients

- ☐ **Cucumber:** 1 unit.
- ☐ **Bitter melon (Cundeamor):** 1 unit.
- ☐ **Chayote:** ½ unit.
- ☐ **Cherries:** ½ cup.
- ☐ **Lemon:** juice of one (1) Lemon (optional).
- ☐ **Water:** 250 ml.

RECOMMENDED TIME TO DRINK

- 10:00 am - 10:30 am
- 4:00 pm - 4:30 pm

You can prepare this Normoglycemic Juice early, carry it to work in a thermos, and drink one or two glasses whenever you feel hungry.

PREPARATION METHOD

1. Thoroughly wash all the ingredients.

2. If preferred, peel the Cucumber and Chayote.

3. Cut the ends off the Bitter melon, cut it in half, then scoop out the seeds with a spoon and discard them. Finally, cut it into small pieces.

4. Place all the ingredients in a blender and blend until the mixture is smooth.

5. Add an ice cube at the end so you can consume it at a pleasant temperature, never cold.

PREPARATION TIME

10 minutes

IMPORTANT NOTES

1. If you are allergic to any component suggested in the recipe, simply do not add it to the preparation.

2. All ingredients should be "to your taste," without forcing the doses.

3. I suggest drinking the juice with a straw, taking a sip every 30 seconds, so it's not unpleasant.

4. If you have a restriction on daily fluid intake due to a condition like Heart or Renal Failure, you should only prepare the amount of Juice according to your doctor's recommendation.

#iamfreeofcomplications

SHOT
immune-boosting

Ingredients

- [ ] **Apple Cider Vinegar:** 1 teaspoon
- [ ] **Própolis:** 5 drops
- [ ] **Lemon:** juice of 1 unit
- [ ] **Mineral Water:** 250 ml

 PREPARATION METHOD

1. In a 300ml glass, place 1 teaspoon of Apple Cider Vinegar.
2. Add the Mineral Water.
3. Add 5 drops of Propolis.
4. Add the juice of 1 Lemon.

PREPARATION TIME

01 minute

⏰ RECOMMENDED TIME

- Drink 10 minutes before Lunch and Dinner for 30 days.

🍴 HOW TO START TAKING IT

- **1st day:** prepare only ½ teaspoon of Apple Cider Vinegar and Propolis in a glass of water.

- **2nd day:** prepare only ½ teaspoon of Apple Cider Vinegar and Propolis in a glass of water.

- **3rd day:** prepare 1 teaspoon of Apple Cider Vinegar and Propolis in a glass of water.

🍴 HOW TO CONSUME THE SHOT

- Drink with a straw and slowly, 1 sip every 1 minute until the entire glass is consumed.

It's important to consider these contraindications and side effects before incorporating Apple Cider Vinegar into your diet. If in doubt, it is advisable to consult a health professional for guidance.

✏️ IMPORTANT NOTES

1. If you have an allergy or any adverse reaction to Apple Cider Vinegar or Propolis, do not include it in the shot.

2. Always dilute the Apple Cider Vinegar in a glass of water. Drinking it pure can damage the throat and wear down dental enamel.

3. You can add a pinch of Cinnamon to help reduce the sour taste of the Vinegar, and if you don't like it, prepare the shot only with Propolis, Lemon, and Mineral Water.

4. Excessive intake of Apple Cider Vinegar can cause gastrointestinal discomfort, such as abdominal pain, nausea, vomiting, and diarrhea.

5. You may experience a burning sensation in the throat due to the acidity of Apple Cider Vinegar.

6. Use unpasteurized Apple Cider Vinegar instead of filtered products. The unpasteurized product contains probiotics that aid digestion.

#iamfreeofcomplications

whole grain rice with CHICKPEAS

Ingredients

- ☐ **Whole Grain Rice:** 2 cups
- ☐ **Chickpeas:** ½ cup
- ☐ **Onion:** 1 unit, finely chopped
- ☐ **Garlic:** 2 cloves, finely chopped
- ☐ **Green (or red) Pepper:** ½ unit
- ☐ **Ora pro nobis (Pereskia aculeata):** 5 leaves
- ☐ **Water:** 3 ½ - 4 cups
- ☐ **Sea Salt (or coarse unrefined salt):** 2 pinches

 PREPARATION METHOD

1. Wash and soak the Chickpeas for a few hours, or overnight.

2. Cook the Chickpeas before cooking the Whole Grain Rice, as follows:

- ■ Place the Chickpeas in a pressure cooker.

- ■ Add enough water to cover the layer of Chickpeas.

- ■ Slowly bring to a boil and cover the pot after 10-15 minutes (do not put the lid on the pot at the beginning).

- ■ Cook on low heat for 1 hour or more until the Chickpeas are 75% cooked.

- ■ As the Chickpeas expand and the water evaporates, gently add more water, letting it run down the sides of the pot to maintain the liquid level until the Chickpeas soften.

PREPARATION TIME

60 minutes

3. Let the Chickpeas cool.

4. Add the Whole Grain Rice to the Chickpeas along with its cooking water, Sea Salt, and the other ingredients in the pressure cooker and stir them.

5. The cooking water from the Chickpeas counts as part of the total water in the recipe.

6. Pressure cook for 40-50 minutes.

7. Once the Whole Grain Rice is done, remove the pot from the heat and let the pressure release naturally (about 5 minutes).

8. Remove the pressure cooker lid, and let the Whole Grain Rice with Chickpeas rest for a few minutes so the grain does not stick to the bottom of the pot.

9. Serve the Whole Grain Rice with Chickpeas on a dish, if possible, using a wooden serving utensil.

10. Garnish the Whole Grain Rice with Chickpeas by adding Carrot, Broccoli, and Parsley to taste.

11. Don't forget to sprinkle Flaxseed, Chia, and Sesame (preferably powdered) on top of the Whole Grain Rice, Vegetable Salads, Soups, etc.

 IMPORTANT NOTES

1. If you are allergic to any component suggested in the recipe, simply do not add it to the preparation.

2. You can eat as much as you want until you feel satisfied.

3. Soaking Whole Grain Rice for a few hours, or overnight, can make it more digestible.

4. Each cup of raw Whole Grain Rice yields, on average, 3 cups of cooked rice.

5. Leftover cooked Whole Grain Rice can be kept out of the refrigerator for 24 hours in a wooden bowl, covered with a bamboo mat or a cotton towel. However, if the environment is very humid or hot, store it in the refrigerator in a sealed container.

6. Reheat Whole Grain Rice using a steamer or place it in a pan, add a little water, cover, and heat for a few minutes.

7. Always, absolutely always, consult your doctor before consuming any new product, especially if you are pregnant, breastfeeding, or have any illness.

#iamfreeofcomplications

whole grain rice with LENTILS

Ingredients

- [ ] **Whole Grain Rice:** 2 cups
- [ ] **Lentils:** ½ cup
- [ ] **Onion:** 1 unit, finely chopped
- [ ] **Garlic:** 2 cloves, finely chopped
- [ ] **Green (or red) Pepper:** ½ unit
- [ ] **Ora pro nobis (Pereskia aculeata):** 5 leaves
- [ ] **Water:** 3 ½ - 4 cups
- [ ] **Sea Salt (or coarse unrefined salt):** 2 pinches

PREPARATION METHOD

1. Wash and soak the Lentils for a few hours, or overnight.

2. Cook the Lentils before cooking the Whole Grain Rice, as follows:

- Place the Lentils in a pressure cooker.
- Add enough water to cover the layer of Lentils.
- Slowly bring to a boil and cover the pot after 10-15 minutes (do not put the lid on the pot at the beginning).
- Cook on low heat for 1 hour or more until the Lentils are 75% cooked.
- As the Lentils expand and water evaporates, gently add more water, letting it run down the sides of the pot to maintain the liquid level until the Lentils soften.

PREPARATION TIME

60
minutes

3. Let the Lentils cool.

4. Add the Whole Grain Rice to the Lentils along with its cooking water, Sea Salt, and the other ingredients in the pressure cooker and stir them.

5. The cooking water from the Lentils counts as part of the total water in the recipe.

6. Pressure cook for 40-50 minutes.

7. Once the Whole Grain Rice is done, remove the pot from the heat and let the pressure release naturally (about 5 minutes).

8. Remove the pressure cooker lid, and let the Whole Grain Rice rest for a few minutes so the grain does not stick to the bottom of the pot.

9. Serve the Whole Grain Rice with Lentils on a dish, if possible, using a wooden serving utensil.

10. Garnish the Whole Grain Rice with Lentils by adding Carrot, Broccoli, and Parsley to taste.

11. Don't forget to sprinkle Flaxseed, Chia, and Sesame (preferably powdered) on top of the Whole Grain Rice, Vegetable Salads, Soups, etc.

 IMPORTANT NOTES

1. If you are allergic to any component suggested in the recipe, simply do not add it to the preparation.

2. You can eat as much as you want until you feel satisfied.

3. Soaking Whole Grain Rice for a few hours, or overnight, can make it more digestible.

4. Each cup of raw Whole Grain Rice yields, on average, 3 cups of cooked rice.

5. Leftover cooked Whole Grain Rice can be kept out of the refrigerator for 24 hours in a wooden bowl, covered with a bamboo mat or a cotton towel. However, if the environment is very humid or hot, store it in the refrigerator in a sealed container.

6. Reheat Whole Grain Rice using a steamer or place it in a pan, add a little water, cover, and heat for a few minutes.

7. Always, absolutely always, consult your doctor before consuming any new product, especially if you are pregnant, breastfeeding, or have any illness.

#iamfreeofcomplications

CORN

whole grain rice with

Ingredients

- ☐ **Whole Grain Rice:** 2 cups
- ☐ **Corn (kernels):** 1 cup
- ☐ **Onion:** 1 unit, finely chopped
- ☐ **Garlic:** 2 cloves, finely chopped
- ☐ **Green (or red) Pepper:** ½ unit
- ☐ **Ora pro nobis (Pereskia aculeata):** 5 leaves
- ☐ **Water:** 3 ½ - 4 cups
- ☐ **Sea Salt (or coarse unrefined salt):** 2 pinches

PREPARATION METHOD

1. Thoroughly wash the grains and Whole Grain Rice and place them in a pressure cooker.

2. Put the pot on the heat, and when the water is hot, add Sea Salt with the other ingredients and stir them.

3. Place the lid on and bring to pressure.

4. Cook for about 45-50 minutes.

5. Remove the pressure cooker lid and let the Whole Grain Rice rest for a few minutes so the grain does not stick to the bottom of the pot.

6. Serve the Whole Grain Rice with Corn on a dish, if possible, using a wooden serving utensil.

7. Serve on a plate and garnish the Whole Grain Rice with Corn presentation by adding Carrot, Broccoli, and Parsley to taste.

8. Don't forget to sprinkle Flaxseed, Chia, and Sesame (preferably powdered) on top of the Whole Grain Rice, Vegetable Salads, Soups, etc.

IMPORTANT NOTES

1. If you are allergic to any component suggested in the recipe, simply do not add it to the preparation.

2. You can eat as much as you want until you feel satisfied.

3. Soaking Whole Grain Rice for a few hours, or overnight, can make it more digestible.

4. Each cup of raw Whole Grain Rice yields, on average, 3 cups of cooked rice.

5. Leftover cooked Whole Grain Rice can be kept out of the refrigerator for 24 hours in a wooden bowl, covered with a bamboo mat or a cotton towel. However, if the environment is very humid or hot, store it in the refrigerator in a sealed container.

6. Reheat the Whole Grain Rice using a steamer or place it in a pan, add a little water, cover, and heat for a few minutes.

7. Always, absolutely always, consult your doctor before consuming any new product, especially if you are pregnant, breastfeeding, or have any illness.

#iamfreeofcomplications

whole grain rice with
QUINOA

Ingredients

- [ ] **Whole Grain Rice:** 2 cups
- [ ] **Quinoa:** 1 cup
- [ ] **Onion:** 1 unit, finely chopped
- [ ] **Garlic:** 2 cloves, finely chopped
- [ ] **Green (or red) Pepper:** ½ unit
- [ ] **Ora pro nobis (Pereskia aculeata):** 5 leaves
- [ ] **Water:** 3 ½ - 4 cups
- [ ] **Sea Salt (or coarse unrefined salt):** 2 pinches

PREPARATION TIME

60 minutes

PREPARATION METHOD

1. Thoroughly wash the Whole Grain Rice and place it in the pressure cooker.

2. Put the pot on the heat and, when the water is hot, add Sea Salt with the other ingredients and stir them.

3. Place the lid on and bring to pressure.

4. Cook for about 45-50 minutes.

5. Remove the pressure cooker lid and let the Whole Grain Rice rest for a few minutes, so the grain does not stick to the bottom of the pot.

6. Serve the Whole Grain Rice with Quinoa on a dish, if possible, using a wooden serving utensil.

7. Serve on a plate and garnish the Whole Grain Rice with Quinoa presentation by adding Carrot, Broccoli, and Parsley to taste.

8. Don't forget to sprinkle Flaxseed, Chia, and Sesame (preferably powdered) on top of the Whole Grain Rice, Vegetable Salads, Soups, etc.

 IMPORTANT NOTES

1. If you are allergic to any component suggested in the recipe, simply do not add it to the preparation.

2. You can eat as much as you want until you feel satisfied.

3. Soaking Whole Grain Rice for a few hours, or overnight, can make it more digestible.

4. Each cup of raw Whole Grain Rice yields, on average, 3 cups of cooked rice.

5. Leftover cooked Whole Grain Rice can be kept out of the refrigerator for 24 hours in a wooden bowl, covered with a bamboo mat or a cotton towel. However, if the environment is very humid or hot, store it in the refrigerator in a sealed container.

6. Reheat the Whole Grain Rice using a steamer or place it in a pan, add a little water, cover, and heat for a few minutes.

7. Always, absolutely always, consult your doctor before consuming any new product, especially if you are pregnant, breastfeeding, or have any illness.

#iamfreeofcomplications

whole grain rice with

MILLET *or* BARLEY

Ingredients

- [ ] **Whole Grain Rice:** 2 cups
- [ ] **Millet or Barley:** 1 cup
- [ ] **Onion:** 1 unit, finely chopped
- [ ] **Garlic:** 2 cloves, finely chopped
- [ ] **Green (or red) Pepper:** ½ unit
- [ ] **Ora pro nobis (Pereskia aculeata):** 5 leaves
- [ ] **Water:** 3 ½ - 4 cups
- [ ] **Sea Salt (or coarse unrefined salt):** 2 pinches

PREPARATION TIME

60 minutes

PREPARATION METHOD

1. Thoroughly wash the Whole Grain Rice and place it in the pressure cooker.

2. Put the pot on the heat and, when the water is hot, add Sea Salt with the other ingredients and stir them.

3. Place the lid on and bring to pressure.

4. Cook for about 45-50 minutes.

5. Remove the pressure cooker lid and let the Whole Grain Rice rest for a few minutes so the grain does not stick to the bottom of the pot.

6. Serve the Whole Grain Rice with Millet on a dish, if possible, using a wooden serving utensil.

7. Serve on a plate and garnish the Whole Grain Rice with Millet or Barley presentation by adding Carrot, Broccoli, and Parsley to taste.

8. Don't forget to sprinkle Flaxseed, Chia, and Sesame (preferably powdered) on top of the Whole Grain Rice, Vegetable Salads, Soups, etc.

 IMPORTANT NOTES

1. If you are allergic to any component suggested in the recipe, simply do not add it to the preparation.

2. You can eat as much as you want until you feel satisfied.

3. Soaking Whole Grain Rice for a few hours, or overnight, can make it more digestible.

4. Each cup of raw Whole Grain Rice yields, on average, 3 cups of cooked rice.

5. Leftover cooked Whole Grain Rice can be kept out of the refrigerator for 24 hours in a wooden bowl, covered with a bamboo mat or a cotton towel. However, if the environment is very humid or hot, store it in the refrigerator in a sealed container.

6. Reheat the Whole Grain Rice using a steamer or place it in a pan, add a little water, cover, and heat for a few minutes.

7. Always, absolutely always, consult your doctor before consuming any new product, especially if you are pregnant, breastfeeding, or have any illness.

#iamfreeofcomplications

steamed VEGETABLES

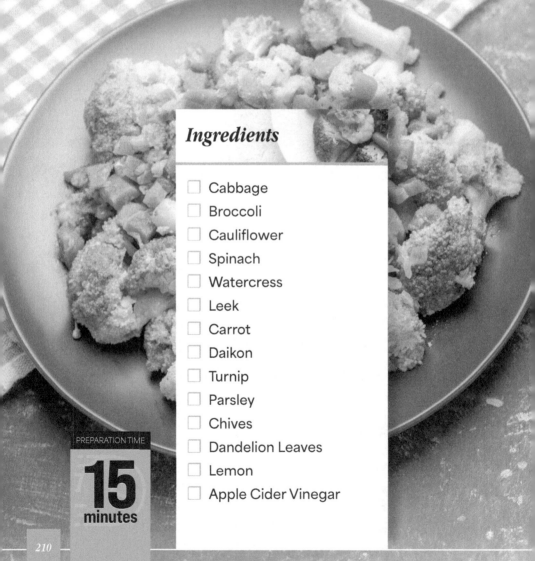

Ingredients

- [ ] Cabbage
- [ ] Broccoli
- [ ] Cauliflower
- [ ] Spinach
- [ ] Watercress
- [ ] Leek
- [ ] Carrot
- [ ] Daikon
- [ ] Turnip
- [ ] Parsley
- [ ] Chives
- [ ] Dandelion Leaves
- [ ] Lemon
- [ ] Apple Cider Vinegar

PREPARATION TIME

15 minutes

PREPARATION METHOD

1. Wash the vegetables thoroughly with plenty of water and chop them.

2. Place the vegetables in a small amount of water, about ½ inch, in a steamer.

3. Cover and simmer or steam for 2-3 minutes, depending on the texture of the vegetables.

4. Quickly place in a bowl to prevent overcooking.

5. Dress with 2 tablespoons of Apple Cider Vinegar, a pinch of salt, and the juice of 1 Lemon.

IMPORTANT NOTES

1. It is not necessary to buy all the vegetables; a combination of 4 is already optimal.

2. Vegetables should have a bright and crunchy color.

3. Wait until the water is completely boiling before placing the vegetables.

4. You may add a few drops of Shoyu at the end of cooking.

5. When boiling, do not cover the pot with a lid or the vegetables will lose their bright green color.

6. There is no restriction on the amount you can eat; that is, you can eat until you feel satisfied.

7. It is not recommended to prepare Cucumber and Tomato in Vegetable Salads, as they are fruits.

#iamfreeofcomplications

stew BARLEY

Ingredients

- [ ] **Barley:** 1 cup
- [ ] **Corn kernels:** 1 cup
- [ ] **Onion:** 1 unit, finely chopped
- [ ] **Garlic:** 2 cloves, finely chopped
- [ ] **Leek:** to taste, finely chopped
- [ ] **Cabbage:** to taste, finely chopped
- [ ] **Carrot:** 1 unit, sliced
- [ ] **Spinach:** to taste
- [ ] **Shiitake mushroom:** 1 unit, finely chopped
- [ ] **Green or red pepper:** ½, finely chopped
- [ ] **Ora pro nobis (Pereskia aculeata):** 5 leaves
- [ ] **Shoyu:** to taste
- [ ] **Water:** 5-6 cups
- [ ] **Sea Salt (or coarse unrefined salt):** 1 pinch

PREPARATION METHOD

1. Thoroughly wash all ingredients.

2. Layer the vegetables in the pot, starting with the onions at the bottom, then the corn, and finally the barley.

3. Gently cook until the barley is done (about 45 minutes).

4. Add Shoyu to taste towards the end of cooking.

5. Serve on a plate and garnish with chives and parsley to taste.

6. Don't forget to sprinkle Flaxseed, Chia, and Sesame (preferably powdered) on top of the Whole Grain Rice, Vegetable Salads, Soups, etc.

PREPARATION TIME

60 minutes

 IMPORTANT NOTES

1. If you are allergic to any component suggested in the recipe, simply do not add it to the preparation.

2. You can eat as much as you want until you feel satisfied.

3. Always, absolutely always, consult your doctor before consuming any new product, especially if you are pregnant, breastfeeding, or have any illness.

#iamfreeofcomplications

Soup
LENTIL

Ingredients

- ☐ **Green or brown lentils:** 1 cup
- ☐ **Onion:** 1 unit, finely chopped
- ☐ **Garlic:** 2 cloves, finely chopped
- ☐ **Leek:** to taste, finely chopped
- ☐ **Cabbage:** to taste, finely chopped
- ☐ **Carrot:** 1 unit, sliced
- ☐ **Spinach:** to taste
- ☐ **Shiitake mushroom:** 1 unit, finely chopped
- ☐ **Green or red pepper:** ½, finely chopped
- ☐ **Ora pro nobis (Pereskia aculeata):** 5 leaves
- ☐ **Shoyu:** to taste
- ☐ **Water:** 5-6 cups
- ☐ **Sea Salt (or coarse unrefined salt):** 1 pinch

PREPARATION METHOD

1. Thoroughly wash all ingredients.

2. Place the chopped onions in a layer at the bottom of the pot, followed by the carrots, and then the lentils on top.

3. Add the water and a pinch of Sea Salt.

4. Bring to a boil, then reduce to a low simmer, cover, and cook for 45 minutes.

5. Add the parsley, the rest of the Sea Salt, and simmer for another 10-15 minutes or until done.

6. For flavor, a little bit of Shoyu can be added at the end of cooking.

7. Serve on a plate and garnish with chives and parsley to taste.

8. Don't forget to sprinkle Flaxseed, Chia, and Sesame (preferably powdered) on top of the Whole Grain Rice, Vegetable Salads, Soups, etc.

PREPARATION TIME

60
minutes

 IMPORTANT NOTES

1. If you are allergic to any component suggested in the recipe, simply do not add it to the preparation.

2. You can eat as much as you want until you feel satisfied.

3. Always, absolutely always, consult your doctor before consuming any new product, especially if you are pregnant, breastfeeding, or have any illness.

#iamfreeofcomplications

215

Soup
CORN

Ingredients

- [ ] **Fresh corn:** 2 cups
- [ ] **Celery:** 1 stalk, diced
- [ ] **Onion:** 1 unit, finely chopped
- [ ] **Garlic:** 2 cloves, finely chopped
- [ ] **Leek:** to taste, finely chopped
- [ ] **Cabbage:** to taste, finely chopped
- [ ] **Carrot:** 1 unit, sliced
- [ ] **Spinach:** to taste
- [ ] **Shiitake mushroom:** 1 unit, finely chopped
- [ ] **Corn kernels:** 1 cup
- [ ] **Green or red pepper:** ½, finely chopped
- [ ] **Ora pro nobis (Pereskia aculeata):** 5 leaves
- [ ] **Watercress and chives:** to taste
- [ ] **Shoyu:** to taste
- [ ] **Water:** 5-6 cups
- [ ] **Sea Salt (or coarse unrefined salt):** 1 pinch

PREPARATION METHOD

1. Thoroughly wash all ingredients.

2. Separate the corn kernels from the cob with the help of a knife.

3. Place the Celery, Onion, Corn, and the rest of the ingredients in a pot.

4. Add water and a pinch of Sea Salt.

5. When it starts to boil, lower the flame, cover, and simmer until the Corn and Celery are soft.

6. Add the rest of the Sea Salt and Shoyu to taste.

7. Serve on a plate and garnish with Chives, Watercress, and Parsley to taste.

8. Don't forget to sprinkle Flaxseed, Chia, and Sesame (preferably powdered) on top of the Whole Grain Rice, Vegetable Salads, Soups, etc.

PREPARATION TIME

60
minutes

✎ **IMPORTANT NOTES**

1. If you are allergic to any component suggested in the recipe, simply do not add it to the preparation.

2. You can eat as much as you want until you feel satisfied.

3. Always, absolutely always, consult your doctor before consuming any new product, especially if you are pregnant, breastfeeding, or have any illness.

#iamfreeofcomplications

Soup MISO

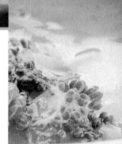

Ingredients

60 minutes

- ☐ **Any variety of Barley Miso**
- ☐ **Corn kernels:** 1 cup
- ☐ **Dry Wakame:** 1 piece of 2 inches by ½ inch
- ☐ **Celery:** 1 stalk, diced
- ☐ **Onion:** 1 unit, finely chopped
- ☐ **Garlic:** 2 cloves, finely chopped
- ☐ **Leek:** to taste, finely chopped
- ☐ **Cabbage:** to taste, finely chopped
- ☐ **Carrot:** 1 unit, sliced
- ☐ **Shiitake mushroom:** 1 unit, finely chopped
- ☐ **Green or red pepper:** ½, finely chopped
- ☐ **Ora pro nobis (Pereskia aculeata):** 5 leaves
- ☐ **Shoyu:** to taste
- ☐ **Water:** 6 cups
- ☐ **Sea Salt (or coarse unrefined salt):** 1 pinch

PREPARATION METHOD

1. Thoroughly wash all ingredients.

2. Soak the Wakame for 5 minutes and cut it into small pieces.

3. Add Wakame to the water and bring to a boil.

4. Add the chopped onions and the rest of the ingredients to the hot broth and boil for 3-5 minutes until the onions are soft and edible, then reduce the flame.

5. Dilute the Miso, ½ or one (1) teaspoon for each cup of broth, in 1 liter of water, add to the soup, and simmer for 3-4 minutes on low heat to prevent the Miso from boiling.

6. Garnish with finely chopped chives and parsley before serving.

7. Don't forget to sprinkle Flaxseed, Chia, and Sesame (preferably powdered) on top of the Whole Grain Rice, Vegetable Salads, Soups, etc.

 IMPORTANT NOTES

1. If you are allergic to any component suggested in the recipe, simply do not add it to the preparation.

2. You can eat as much as you want until you feel satisfied.

3. Make sure to simmer the soup for 3-4 minutes after adding the Miso. Miso should not be boiled as it loses its healthy properties.

4. For variety, you can use other types of aged Miso for more than 2 years (Soy or Rice), occasionally.

5. Vary the vegetables daily. Some combinations are Onions-Tofu, Onions-Zucchini, Common Cabbage-Carrots; and Daikon Roots-Leaves.

6. Frequently include leafy vegetables like Kale, Collards, Watercress, etc., being careful to add them at the end of the preparation to avoid long cooking times.

7. Leftover grains or beans from previous meals can be used to make a thicker soup.

8. For the best effects, try to prepare Miso Soup each time it is to be consumed and do not use the leftover from late in the day or avoid leaving it overnight.

9. Always, absolutely always, consult your doctor before consuming any new product, especially if you are pregnant, breastfeeding, or have any illness.

#iamfreeofcomplications

MILLET

and sweet vegetable soup

50
minutes

Ingredients

- [ ] **Millet:** 1 cup
- [ ] **Corn kernels:** 1 cup
- [ ] **Celery:** 1 stalk, diced
- [ ] **Zucchini:** ½ cup, finely chopped
- [ ] **Cauliflower:** to taste, finely chopped
- [ ] **Broccoli:** to taste, finely chopped
- [ ] **Carrots:** ½ cup, finely chopped
- [ ] **Cabbage:** ½ cup, finely chopped
- [ ] **Onion:** ½, finely chopped
- [ ] **Wakame:** 1 piece of 1 inch
- [ ] **Shiitake mushroom:** 1 small piece
- [ ] **Shoyu:** a few drops to taste
- [ ] **Chives or Parsley:** to taste
- [ ] **Water:** 6 cups
- [ ] **Sea Salt (or coarse unrefined salt):** 1 pinch

PREPARATION METHOD

1. Thoroughly wash all ingredients.

2. Wash the Millet and mix with the mentioned ingredients except for the seasonings.

3. Add 3 times more water than the ingredients and a pinch of salt.

4. Bring to a boil, then reduce the flame and simmer for about 30 minutes, until cooked.

5. Towards the end of cooking, lightly season with a few drops of shoyu and simmer for another 3-4 minutes.

6. Garnish with finely chopped chives and parsley before serving.

7. Don't forget to sprinkle Flaxseed, Chia, and Sesame (preferably powdered) on top of the Whole Grain Rice, Vegetable Salads, Soups, etc.

 IMPORTANT NOTES

1. If you are allergic to any component suggested in the recipe, simply do not add it to the preparation.

2. You can eat as much as you want until you feel satisfied.

3. Always, absolutely always, consult your doctor before consuming any new product, especially if you are pregnant, breastfeeding, or have any illness.

#iamfreeofcomplications

olive oil and lemon SHOT

Olive Oil is a vegetable oil obtained from the fruit of the Olive tree (Olea europaea), native to the Mediterranean region. This oil is highly valued for its flavor, nutritional properties, and multiple uses, both in cooking and in cosmetics and medicine.

Especially the unrefined Extra Virgin Olive Oil is known to be a source of monounsaturated fats, particularly oleic acid. It also contains antioxidants such as polyphenols and vitamin E, which can offer health benefits.

BENEFITS OF EXTRA VIRGIN OLIVE OIL

- **Cardiovascular Benefits:** regular consumption contributes to cardiovascular health as monounsaturated fats help to reduce LDL cholesterol ("bad cholesterol") and improve heart health.

- **Natural Antioxidant:** the polyphenols present in Olive Oil have antioxidant properties that help protect the body's cells against damage caused by free radicals.

- **Skin Health:** it is used in skincare products due to its ability to moisturize and soften the skin. It has also been associated with reducing inflammation and promoting healing.

- **Disease Prevention:** some studies suggest that the consumption of Extra Virgin Olive Oil may be associated with a lower incidence of chronic diseases, such as heart disease and type 2 diabetes mellitus.

- **Digestion and Nutrient Absorption:** it promotes digestion and absorption of fat-soluble nutrients due to its content of healthy fats.

 RECOMMENDED TIME

- **10:00 pm.** Always before sleeping and after the Normoglycemic Tea.

 HOW TO CONSUME

- Drink it in one gulp; there's no need to keep the mixture in your mouth.

 PREPARATION METHOD

In a glass, place a tablespoon of unrefined Extra Virgin Olive Oil with the juice of one Lemon and stir the mixture.

 IMPORTANT NOTES

1. If you have a known allergy to Olive Oil or Lemon, do not consume them.

2. It's important to choose high-quality Olive Oil, preferably unrefined Extra Virgin, as it retains more nutrients and flavor compared to other varieties.

3. This shot may be unpleasant to the palate, so I suggest you take it in one gulp, without "thinking twice," or you can add a pinch of honey, as long as it is proven that honey ingestion does not increase your blood sugar levels.

#iamfreeofcomplications

223

MENTAL *reprogramming*

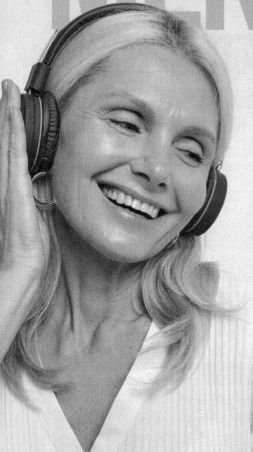

AUDIO OR VIDEO

It's a powerful tool used to positively influence a person's thoughts, behavior, and emotions through specific messages.

These resources are often indicated to help you change negative thought patterns, promote self-confidence, reduce stress, improve self-image, and encourage healthy habits. Benefits:

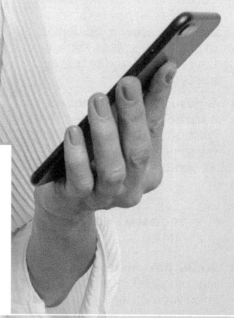

 PROPOSAL

The audio we recommend can be found on the internet as: "Direct to Your Subconscious Mind" - "I AM" Affirmations for Success, Wealth, and Happiness Or any other audio that you like.

BENEFÍCIOS

1. Reduction of Stress and Anxiety: chronic stress can negatively affect diabetes control. Listening to a Mental Reprogramming audio helps reduce stress and anxiety and has a positive impact on blood sugar levels.

2. Adherence to Treatment: listening to positive and motivating affirmations related to diabetes management will increase the motivation to follow the Treatment Plan.

3. Promotion of Healthy Habits: mental Reprogramming audios will help you change negative thought patterns and promote the adoption of healthy habits.

4. Strengthening Self-esteem and Confidence: diabetes mellitus can affect self-image. Positive messages in Mental Reprogramming audios contribute to improving self-esteem and confidence in the ability to reverse the damage of the disease.

5. Improvement of Glycemic Control: if you firmly believe in your ability to control diabetes and adopt a Healthy Lifestyle daily, it is more likely that you will maintain blood glucose levels within normal ranges.

6. Promotion of Relaxation and Overall Well-being: the audios include relaxation techniques that will help you reduce blood pressure, improve sleep quality, and promote a general state of well-being.

7. Emotional Support: listening to supportive and understanding messages through Mental Reprogramming audios will help you deal with emotions related to the disease and feel less isolated.

ADVICE FROM DR. QUESADA

If you have an Alexa device, or any other device that allows you to set an alarm with a personalized audio, I suggest you do it so that you wake up with a Mental Reprogramming audio, making it easier to start your daily routine.

#iamfreeofcomplications

Posture correction and hypopressive
EXERCISES

Knees to Chest ▪ Hip Rotation ▪ Hip Lift

These are techniques used to improve posture and strengthen the core muscles (abdominal and lumbar area) through breathing and specific muscle activation.

 BENEFITS

1. Improved Posture: they help to correctly align the spine, reducing tension and pressure on the back, neck, and shoulders, thus improving overall posture.

2. Intestinal Regulation: they activate the deep abdominal muscles and favor breathing control, which improves the gastrointestinal system's functioning. This activation helps stimulate intestinal peristalsis and favor intestinal regularity, thus reducing constipation and improving overall digestion.

3. Increased Energy and Stamina: these exercises typically involve deep and controlled breathing, increasing tissue oxygenation, which in turn increases sexual disposition and vitality.

4. Eliminates Fluid Retention: hypopressive exercises, focused on contracting and strengthening core muscles, stimulate the lymphatic and circulatory systems. This helps reduce fluid retention, improving circulation, and facilitating the elimination of toxins and stagnant fluids in tissues.

5. Intra-abdominal Viscera Massage: the technique of hypopressive exercises consists of the controlled contraction and relaxation of abdominal and pelvic floor muscles. This movement functions as a kind of gentle massage of the intra-abdominal viscera, stimulating blood circulation and the proper functioning of internal organs.

EXERCISE 1

KNEES TO CHEST

DURATION

01
minute

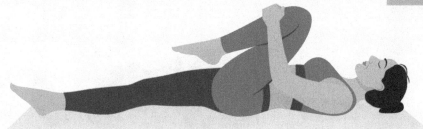

STARTING POSITION

On the bed, after waking up, in the supine position, bend your knees with your feet resting on the bed in a pyramid shape, so your knees point towards the ceiling.

MOVEMENT

1. Perform several deep breaths before starting.

2. Grab your right knee with both hands and slowly pull it towards your chest while taking a deep breath. Without forcing the movement, try to touch your chin with your knee.

3. Hold the knee close to the chest for 5 seconds, contracting the abdominal muscles and the left leg slightly bent.

4. Then return to the starting position while making a deep exhalation.

5. Now repeat the same operation with the left leg and then with both legs together.

IMPORTANT NOTES

1. You should feel the muscles stretching but not pain.

2. Do not perform this exercise if it causes or increases pain in the back or any part of the body.

3. Do not perform this exercise if you have any contraindications such as disc hernia, spinal problems, etc.

4. Before starting any exercise program, you should consult with your doctor.

#iamfreeofcomplications

227

DURATION

01
minute

EXERCISE 2
HIP ROTATION

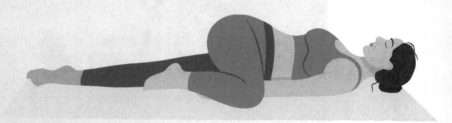

STARTING POSITION

On the bed, after having performed the previous exercise, remain in a supine position, with knees bent and feet in contact with the bed. Place your arms stretched out on either side of your body in a T position relative to the body.

 MOVEMENT

Keeping the upper part of the body straight, let your bent knees fall to one side and rotate the torso to the opposite side. This entire movement should be accompanied by a deep exhalation. Hold this position for 5 seconds with the shoulders supported on the bed. Return to the first position, taking a deep breath in and repeat the exercise for the other side.

IMPORTANT NOTES

1. You should feel the muscles stretching but not pain.

2. Do not perform this exercise if it causes or increases pain in the back or any part of the body.

3. This is one of the back stretches that you can also perform twice a day, and between two or three repetitions.

4. Do not perform this exercise if you have any contraindications such as disc hernia, spinal problems, etc.

5. Before starting any exercise program, you should consult with your doctor.

EXERCISE 3
HIP LIFT

DURATION
01
minute

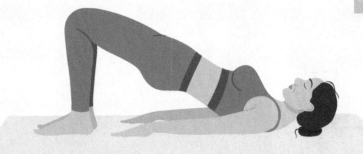

STARTING POSITION

After performing the previous exercise, remain in a supine position, with knees bent and feet in contact with the bed. Place your arms stretched out on either side of your body.

▷ MOVEMENT

Tightening the abdomen and glutes, lift the hips to form a straight line from the knees to the shoulders, and inhale deeply, "sucking" the abdomen inward and "squeezing" the abdominal viscera. Try to maintain this position and breathe deeply three times, then return to the starting position and repeat the exercise.

IMPORTANT NOTES

1. You should feel the muscles stretching but not pain.

2. Do not perform the exercise if it causes or increases pain in the back or leg.

3. Do not perform this exercise if you have any contraindications such as disc hernia, spinal problems, etc. Before starting any exercise program, you should consult with your doctor.

#iamfreeofcomplications

Breathing
EXER
CISES

Breathing exercises, accompanied by music or relaxing sounds, are specific techniques used to control and improve the way we breathe.

These exercises can have a number of health benefits, including stimulating body detoxification and promoting health recovery.

Here is a list of some of the benefits of breathing exercises related to body detoxification and health:

BENEFITS

- **Improved Oxygenation:** deep breathing exercises help bring more oxygen to the body's cells, which can increase the efficiency of detoxification processes.

- **Stress Reduction:** deep and controlled breathing can reduce stress levels, which in turn can promote a stronger immune system and better detoxification capacity.

- **Improved Circulation:** breathing exercises can improve blood circulation, which can help eliminate toxins and improve overall health.

- **Strengthened Immune System:** regular practice of breathing exercises can strengthen the immune system, which can help the body better defend against toxins and diseases.

- **Reduction of Inflammation:** chronic inflammation is related to many diseases. Deep breathing can help reduce inflammation, which can contribute to health recovery.

- **Increased Energy and Vitality:** more efficient breathing can increase energy levels and help the body function more effectively in eliminating toxins.

- **Improved Digestion:** deep and relaxing breathing can aid digestion, which can influence the proper elimination of wastes and toxins from the body.

- **Promotion of Relaxation:** deep relaxation through conscious breathing can stimulate the release of health-beneficial hormones and aid in the recovery of various conditions.

- **Stimulation of the Lymphatic System:** deep and conscious breathing can help move lymph through the lymphatic system, which can aid in the elimination of toxins from the body.

- **Support for Mental Health:** breathing exercises can also be beneficial for mental health, reducing anxiety and depression, which in turn can improve overall health.

To contribute to the body detoxification process and obtain the mentioned benefits, I recommend listening to the video that can be found on the internet as:

- Guided Wim Hof Breathing Exercises.

- Or any breathing exercise that you prefer.

#iamfreeofcomplications

Sea Salt
FOOT BATH

With this simple yet powerful procedure, you can quickly lower blood sugar levels, in addition to having other powerful therapeutic effects.

The Sea Salt Foot Bath - unrefined - also known as a "Foot Bath," is an ancestral therapy passed down from generation to generation that promotes the elimination of toxins from the body.

This simple yet powerful therapy should be applied periodically to maintain health, as its therapeutic effects are proven both physically and mentally, as well as spiritually.

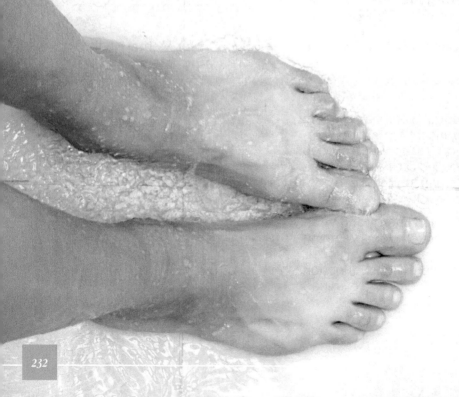

HISTORY

It is estimated that this therapy was already being used six thousand years ago to provide relaxation and body cleansing.

According to traditional Chinese medicine, based on the balance of Yin and Yang polarity, the Foot Bath helps distribute this Yang energy (head) to the cold extremities (Yin energy).

 ## WHY ADD SALT TO THE WATER?

The difference in saline solution concentration between the intra and extracellular environment generates a potential difference (electrical currents) between two spaces, causing changes in cellular activities and, consequently, in tissue aspects, enabling the transmission of electrical current.

There is a variation in conductivity in each tissue of the human body; those with more dissolved ions in their composition are the best.

When we add salts to water, they dissociate forming ions that conduct electricity. By putting the feet in contact with this electrolytic solution, the electrical force generated by the ions dispersed in the water causes the ions from the human body's cells to migrate in the direction of this external force towards attraction or repulsion.

This ionic action can cause significant physiological changes at various levels of the organism: cellular, tissue, organ, and systemic.

#iamfreeofcomplications

THERAPEUTIC EFFECT

With this simple procedure, you can quickly lower blood sugar levels, and also:

- Eliminate toxins from the blood, aiding the body's detoxification process, which further reduces insulin resistance.

- Purify organs such as the brain, kidneys, prostate, liver, reproductive system, and lungs.

- Reduce stress and emotional burdens, controlling anxiety and insomnia.

- Balance counterregulatory hormone levels.

- Activate blood and lymphatic circulation.

- Eliminate edema and fluid retention.

- Reduce pain and inflammation.

- Relax joints, muscles, and bones.

- Strengthen the immune system.

- Prevent varicose veins and thrombosis.

- Alleviate chronic fatigue and facilitate rest.

 INDICATIONS

As therapy to favor detoxification and treatment of any disease.

 PRECAUTIONS

For people with high blood pressure, the water should not be too cold or too hot; it must be lukewarm. It's important to know that preparing the foot bath with lukewarm water can stabilize blood pressure.

 CONTRAINDICATIONS

- Pregnant women;

- People with cancer in a metastatic situation.

SESSIONS
Perform 2 times/day

 RECOMMENDED TIME

7:00 am
9:00 pm

ooo STEPS

1. Boil approximately 3 liters of water with the grated ginger. When it starts to boil, turn off the heat and let it cool slightly until lukewarm.

2. Pour a sufficient amount of lukewarm water (should be between 36°C and 39°C) into the basin, enough to cover the ankles (approximately 3L).

3. Add the Sea Salt and stir the water to dissolve.

4. Now you should immerse your feet in the water for 30 minutes, always ensuring the temperature is comfortable.

5. Wet a small towel in the ginger water and gently massage your legs in a circular motion from the feet up to the knees. Repeat the process for 1 to 3 minutes, avoiding skin trauma.

6. After 30 minutes, remove your feet from the water, dry them with a towel, and put on socks to keep them warm.

 RESOURCES

- **Lukewarm water:** should be between 36°C - 39°C (96.8°F - 102.2°F) and in sufficient quantity (3L).
- **Sea Salt:** 1 cup (you can use coarse unrefined salt).
- **Ginger:** ¼ unit (grated).
- **Basin:** to place the feet.
- **Towel:** to scrub and dry the feet.

 IMPORTANT NOTES

1. It's preferable to use coarse unrefined Sea Salt but, if you don't have this type of salt, you can use any variety.

2. The use of Ginger is optional. If you use it, it enhances the therapeutic effect, but if you don't have ginger, you can do the foot bath with just water and Sea Salt.

3. Remember to drink the Normoglycemic Tea while doing the foot bath.

4. Listen to the Relaxation Audio and practice the Breathing Technique during the 30 minutes of the foot bath.

#iamfreeofcomplications

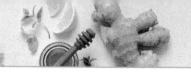

POWERFUL TIPS
for Living a Fulfilling Life

Dear Therapist, we are now reaching the end, and I find it appropriate and necessary to share with you 17 Tips, or Lifestyle Suggestions, to maintain harmony and health.

These suggestions, as he called them, were created by my mentor Rafael Milanés and, with the deference that characterized him, he shared them with me as they are not published in any book or article on the internet.

I invite you to read them with great affection and, above all, to incorporate them into your day-to-day life as a project for a harmonious and healthy life.

LIFESTYLE SUGGESTIONS
By Rafael Milanés Santana

Following these suggestions will contribute to a healthy, peaceful, and orderly life:

1. Maintain the dream and image of health for yourself, others, and the planet.

2. Live each day happily without carrying health worries and remain active and alert both physically and mentally.

3. Be thankful for whatever happens or whoever you meet. Offer thanks before and after each meal.

4. It's better to go to bed before midnight and rise early, especially with the sunrise.

5. Avoid wearing synthetic or woolen clothes directly in contact with the skin. Use cotton (preferably organic and not genetically modified) as much as possible, especially for underwear. Avoid excessive metallic ornaments on fingers, wrists, or neck. Keep ornaments that are elegant and simple.

6. If your strength allows, engage in outdoor activities with simple clothing. Walk between 30 minutes and 1 hour daily preferably on the earth, grass, or beach sand.

7. Maintain order in your house and the surrounding environment.

8. Start and maintain active correspondence with friends and family wishing the best for them. Also, initiate and maintain the best relationships with those around you.

9. Avoid taking long hot baths or showers, as you can lose vitamins and minerals through your skin.

10. Rub your body with a hot, damp towel every morning and every night before going to sleep until the skin reddens. If this is not possible, at least do it on your hands, feet, and respective fingers.

11. Avoid chemically perfumed cosmetics. Use natural preparations or sea salt for tooth care.

12. If your condition allows, stay physically active as part of your daily life by carrying out household chores like scrubbing floors and windows and activities such as yoga, dance, martial arts, or sports.

13. Avoid the use of electrical appliances for cooking and microwave ovens. Convert your kitchen to gas or wood at the first opportunity.

14. Minimize the use of computers, television, cell phones, and other electronic devices that emit artificial electromagnetic energy.

15. Include green plants in your home to refresh and enrich the oxygen content of the air.

16. Anyone can learn to prepare healthy meals. Participate in some part of the food preparation process, whether it be harvesting, buying, processing, cooking the food, or even washing the dishes.

17. Sing a happy song every day.

#iamfreeofcomplications

I'm thrilled to know that you've
made it this far!

I can imagine the peace and assurance you must feel upon discovering a reliable, swift, and 100% effective method to reverse the damage caused by diabetes mellitus, freeing yourself from potential risks and complications.

Your dedication, effort, and commitment are unmatched, so I invite you to embark on this transformative journey with me, and that's why I recommend you always keep this book within reach, so you can consult it frequently. Now that you've discovered the END OF DIABETES MELLITUS method, put it into practice as indicated, and let it become part of your life and your daily routine.

A Special Request

After completing the first 30 days following the method, if you feel that this book has made a difference in your life, I encourage you to share your testimony with other diabetics on social media, especially in Facebook groups.

Sharing your experience with the world, I'm certain, will help me save more lives as there are thousands of people who have lost faith and are losing the battle against diabetes mellitus.

Can I count on you to make a difference in the lives of the sickest and most needy?

I will also be extremely honored if, upon receiving a copy of my book, you ask a family member to take a photo of you with it in your hands and share it on your social media.

You can tag me -*@draldenquesada.es*-, and use **#IAm-FreeOfComplications**, because I want to get to know you and share in your joy.

In this way, in addition to demonstrating your commitment to the universe and our Creator, you will also be motivating thousands of people with diabetes to live free from risks and complications.

and remember

You have a life mission:
To live fully every day, but live with Health.

I hope that each recommendation in this book becomes an endless source of life for you, your family, and the people you love.

the end of DIABETIC

*Have you ever been to the Emergency Services due to **high blood sugar levels** and symptoms?*

*Most diabetic individuals go through this dangerous situation, and that's why I want you to **retake 100% control of your life.***

*My greatest wish is for you to be able to share **joyful moments** again with your family and friends, **without the worry** that acute complications of diabetes mellitus might arise...*

———

By applying what is in this book, you will be able to participate in a birthday party, a gathering, or a family dinner without having to worry about high blood sugar levels.

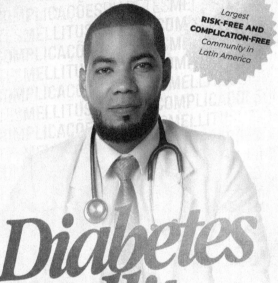

If you're looking to dive deeper into taking care of and recovering your health, you can also find me at:

📷 🐦 ▶️ @draldenquesada.es

WWW.ALDENQUESADA.COM

Follow me on my social networks. I'm sure that together we will learn a great deal about how to live with health and harmony #diseasefree.

"I have come that they may have life, and have it to the full."

JOHN 10:10

LIVE AS FULLY AS POSSIBLE,
but live with health!

Alden J. Quesada